ALIVE!
An Energy
Plan for Life

Rae Hatherton

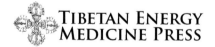
TIBETAN ENERGY
MEDICINE PRESS

Library of Congress Cataloguing-in-Publication Data

ISBN 978-0-9868358-0-3

Design and layout by Steve Stivers
Edited by Andrea Lemieux
Index by Judith Brand

Tibetan Energy Medicine Press
40 Park Road, Suite 206
Toronto, Ontario
Canada
M4W 2N4

Printed and bound in USA

To my teachers—my source

To my clients and friends—my inspiration

Please use this book as a workbook.

I have designed this book with its extended dimensions and extra-large margins to give you space to write your own notes and add information. You are not desecrating this volume by writing in its margins, highlighting, or generally adding to its content. The book is designed for you! It is a life manual and is meant to be used and engaged with rather than just read. Please personalize it and add your unique perspective on the lessons and guidance that I am sharing with you here.

FREE BONUS DOWNLOADS

go to www.alivethebook.com
and put in your purchase information and email address.

CONTENTS

FOREWORD

From the earliest human records in the metaphysical and cosmological systems of the world's great faiths and sacred traditions, it has been acknowledged that levels of reality reflect higher levels: "as above, so below." The human body is prefigured in the spiritual realm and then "clothed" in the physical body here on earth. The purpose of this body sheath, or vehicle, is to provide—for a brief span of years—the opportunity for the Witness, or immortal soul within, to recognize its veritable Divine Essence. Using the five senses, with which this luminous soul is temporarily endowed, the mortal soul is engaged with many trials involving loss of life, cherished ideals, and goods. The mortal soul has been given directives from a sacred system as to how to transform such suffering into recollection or remembrance of its true primordial nature, variously called by the different religions: the Christ-like nature, Fitrah, Buddha-nature, Adama, and so on.

But the physical body—an extension of the spiritual body—must be part of this alchemical transformation. It cannot do so easily if it is not vertically aligned with the spiritual domain it reflects. An analogy might be a plumb line from the crown of one's head descending through the body. As it passes through the various planes/chakras/centers, it reflects the correct way to be, do, or think. For example, in the mind—correct thinking, in the mouth—correct speaking, in the stomach—correct eating, and in the body in general—correct or balanced exercise. If our body is off balance and we do not care for it so that it may function optimally at each level, we are sabotaging its higher spiritual function. If we are to be fully human, all the levels of our being must correspond and work together in order for us to return fully to the Divine Source and fulfill the purpose of our physical manifestation. If we've damaged or do not care for and properly sustain the vehicle with which we are provided for this sacred journey, heedlessness is nothing short of irresponsibility and unconsciousness of the Ultimate Reality.

— Gray Henry, Author,
Publisher, and Friend

PREFACE

I truly love France. Of all the places I have been in the world, it has captured my heart and I feel more at peace there than anywhere else I have been so far.

In the spring of 2010, when I was at my friend's home in the countryside outside Paris, I examined what it was that made me feel so at home, so comforted, and so quiet in my mind. I took a look at the French people, who are famous for being distant and not too likeable; I see this as an inclination to give privacy to others, although others may see it as simply standoffish. I gave an eye to the weather, which was quite cool but not extraordinary for spring in this part of the world. I observed the culture; the ancient and modern architecture; the lands and the *châteaux*; the prettiness of the landscapes neatly drawn with winding roads, well-manicured fields, and *les petits bois* (the little forests). France is famous for its food and wine, which always have their allure, but one can find excellent food and great wine elsewhere in the world.

All of those things are wonderful and in some ways uniquely French—but it is not those external manifestations of order, taste, and beauty that take my heart. As I reduced it down by a process of elimination, I discovered what was truly there: a connection to what is natural, a connection between humanity and nature—an intrinsic song of life sung over centuries of timing with nature, in agriculture and agrarian habits—and an intimate connection with and support of humanity—alive!

France, with its rigid structured social model and culture of farm living, has maintained a life standard that is still connected to the values of nature, those values that have maintained us as a species for thousands of years. It is that connection with the laws of nature that provides all beings with a structure for healing and growth. In most parts of the Western world we have lost that connection. Those values have been eclipsed by a new set of standards and values that are gradually killing us with packaged fast food, stress, fast living, more and more complex lifestyles, technology, and lost morals.

This book is about getting back to the connection to nature and to self, to get in touch with what makes us *sentir bien dans notre peau*, feel good in our skin. The idea for the Plan came to me after my sessions with a doctor in a small town near Geneva, Switzerland, several years ago, and it came together in the French side of Switzerland, and I wrote this book in Geneva and the farmlands of France.

For most of my life, I struggled with metabolism and all the side effects of sluggish endocrine function: hormone imbalance, anemia, heavy periods, issues with digestion and elimination, low blood sugar, miscarriages, and problems with energy and moods. As a natural-health practitioner, and even before that as a layperson constantly in search of solutions, I shared any knowledge

gleaned or newfound fixes with friends and, eventually, with clients. However, nothing really lasted or was efficient enough to handle all of the associated metabolic problems.

Then in 2004 I was visiting a friend in Switzerland who introduced me to a nutritionist in a small town in the beautiful Swiss Alps. Flying to Paris, to Geneva, and then driving for two and a half hours through the mountains to get to the town where this fellow worked made me very committed. For a year, including subsequent visits, I followed the system exactly as prescribed and had very good results. My sluggish system took several months to pick up—a fair amount of time, but I got results. The results stuck and I got turned on. The Swiss nutritionist had combined many modalities into his method, which inspired me to do the same in my practice. Although he had a few unique approaches, most of the modalities were ones I had used previously from other bodies of work I'd studied over the years. As I worked on developing my own set of modalities for the Plan, each experience from my past training and multiple teachers seemed to jump forward and ask to be included in the practical application of the structure of the Plan.

I wrote this book to explain how and why this way of living will work for you. It has worked consistently well for many people over the past five years, and as a bonus, the lifestyle they have adopted has changed them forever. You will see in the testimonials throughout the book that this is not a diet or a cleansing program, but a healing shift in perspective around our connection to food, eating, self-image, and being fully and completely on the road to being alive.

For the first several years of designing the Plan and working with it with clients, I called it the Swissplan, but if anything, it should be called Rae's Plan. However, I have finally settled on Alive! An Energy Plan for Life, and I refer to it as "the Plan" throughout this book. I think everyone would like a plan, a structure, a map, a

direction to follow that works. And it is that. It is a plan that works.

Your results will not be merely metabolic or just in the physical domain, and this is what I hope to communicate in these pages. This map is about being fully and completely and on all levels *alive*. The energy plan that will be described in the following pages will help bring you to life, and *alive* will become your motto, your credo, and what people will notice about you.

It is my sincere wish that there is enough information here to satisfy your need for hows and whys, and to satisfy your mind. This is not a technical book like many other books about lifestyle change; it is a book about a simple practice of living that just works. I hope that it inspires you to have the will—and the courage—to proceed with this energy plan for life and that it brings you success, self-awareness, well-being, and peace.

ACKNOWLEDGMENTS

I wish to thank all my teachers and friends for their invaluable knowledge, which has framed the background for this book. I will name a few, but there are many more who shall go unnamed. Much water has gone under the bridge since I began thinking about this idea, and the teachers have been ever present. I am grateful to Jack, the Tibetan monk who had me remember who I was, introduced me to the nature of mind, and coaxed and cajoled me into admitting I was capable of whatever I truly desired to do for the benefit of all; my present teacher, Sogyal Rinpoche, a constant inspiration, who, in a complicated study of life, makes things clear and simple and inspires one to act; His Holiness the XIVth Dalai Lama, with whom I will spend time as often as possible, basking in his wisdom, dry humor, simplicity, and compassion; Tsoknyi Rinpoche for teaching *lungta* breath and for his quick wit and precise insight; and to my Buddhist dharma sister Ane Sangye Chözom, who selflessly promotes me

inside and outside the sangha. I thank Hanna Kroeger, Bobbi Brooks, Brent Williams, and Lori Wilson, who had me trust the dance of nature and the body.

Thank you to my dear friend Agathe Heurteux and her parents for introducing me to M. Bueschi in a tiny town in the Swiss Alps, where the idea for the Plan was born, and who opened her heart and her houses for me to write in over the years. To my dear friends Pumpkin and Rob Auerbach and the extended Auerbach family, including Summer, Star, and their partners, as well as Noah, Sy, and Minx, Amy and John Peterson, Jack, Lucy, and pets, who support me and empower everything that I do in every way they know possible, and who are not blood relatives, but better. To Jean Elizabeth Grabowski for her faith in my ability to write and for providing me with the first opportunity I had to write in her magazine *Illuminations*. To my friend Terry St. Pierre, who helped me think, articulate, and frame thought, of which she is a master. To Mary Shands for providing a staff and a venue to support a healing retreat at Foxhollow Farm, as well as the many years I had the good fortune to work with her, and for the wonderful connections I made through her that have benefited me to this day. To Virginia Lake and Tom Olien, long-time friends, partners, and always a support. To Gray Henry for her constant spiritual partnership and for sharing her friends and colleagues with me. To Laura Clunie and her gang in the UK for their support and promotion. To Kimberly and Richard May for their friendship and support. To Eunice Ray and the girls from Arbonne. To my herbalist, Jenny Boice, for her wonderful teas and tinctures and her constant support and participation in the work. To Valerie Oxorn and Dot Whitehouse for being my wall—the place where you throw things against to see if they stick. To the managers and the staff of Rainbow Blossom Natural Foods for supporting my work through events and networking, for supporting the Plan as it evolved and Tibetan Acupressure, another heartsong of mine, and for putting up with my endless requests for

my clients.

To my daughter, Arin, who believes in and supports me unconditionally. To David and Fran Hatherton and their children, and to my mother, Margaret Hatherton, for being my family. To my dad, who, although he is a long time passed, inspires me to be the entrepreneurial spirit that I am.

To my many editors, whom I thank for their support, patience, and constructive input, especially Lin Stranberg. I am deeply grateful to Andrea Lemieux, who provided the most crucial editing to the final manuscript.

I thank Steve Stivers, the skilled artisan who designed this book, for his patience and understanding through the many changes this book underwent.

And last but not least, to my clients, who are the inspiration for this book and for my ongoing life and work. I thank them for their perseverance, contribution, and inspiration, in sickness and in health. May their contribution be rewarded with good health and a peaceful mind.

PROLOGUE

Years ago, the lotus flower became the logo for my work in helping people improve their lives. I chose this exquisite flower for its beauty and its symbolic meaning. Arising from murky swamp waters, the lotus is a flower of stainless purity. This echoed something very stirring that I had seen in my life's work. The lotus flower embodies the ability to transform.

Time and again I have witnessed that, as people, we have the power to transform ourselves. We can alter our lives and perspectives and return to that stainless inner purity that is always available to us. Not only that, but we can also survive destructive attitudes and harsh circumstances. Though these experiences are damaging, our resilient spirit can shine through and reclaim our true, pure nature. I have always believed that it is that "coming home" to the purity of self that defines us as human beings.

When we consider the depth of human suffering, the ideas of appearance, weight, and achievement may seem trivial at first. Yet we all know that poor body image and ill health cause the kind of suffering that crushes vitality, damages confidence, and can eventually diminish the spirit. In day-to-day reality, it is like muddy swamp water. Yet, like the lotus, we can grow by reaching through the suffering into the joyful experience of strength and beauty.

It is only natural to dedicate this book to you, my reader, some of whom may be my clients—present, former, or future—as my work with the Plan has always been dedicated to those who have suffered but who are searching to reclaim themselves. It is my hope that my work will alleviate the suffering and expand the minds of those who decide to *listen*. If we truly listen to ourselves, we can find the way to connect with our purest, most authentic essence to come alive again. The goal of this book is to give you the structure and the opportunity to flourish and grow fully into your beautiful lotus self. The Plan will give you the structure to find your body's metabolic balance, balancing your chemistry, and through that become closer to your center. May your transformation give you peace of mind and a settled spirit. And although it seems like a tall order, my wish is that your new-found peace of mind extends its benefit to all beings and creates a ripple effect of peace and joy in the world.

ALIVE! An Energy Plan for Life
What It Is and Why It Works

Alive! An Energy Plan for Life is an integrated system of lifestyle changes designed to shift the body into an efficient creator of energy and well-being. It combines nutrition and food combining, detoxification, living by our body's natural rhythms, breathing, physical exercise, meditation, mindful awareness, and listening. It is designed to improve digestion and protein metabolism, oxygenate the blood, balance neurotransmitters, and maintain healthy blood sugar levels, resulting in a metabolic shift, and thus, a new you!

Eating three meals a day, having an early dinner, and going to bed with the sun (well, a little bit later—10 p.m.) cause the body to reset its biological clock. Learning to breathe Tibetan-style—into the belly— balances the brain's neurotransmitters and brings the focus of energy from the cognitive and emotional centers into the energy center of the body, just below the navel. Food combining reduces the effort required for digestion by increasing enzymatic activity and making assimilation more effective, so energy is released in a more consistent fashion.

Ancient Tibetan metabolic exercises, often referred to as the fountain-of-youth antiaging yoga, stimulate the endocrine organs, which improves hormone function. The result is youthful energy, a feeling of being alive, and spontaneity.

In addition, specifically formulated

herbal teas combined with the stimulation of Tibetan acupressure points on the feet and legs increase circulation, kick-start the metabolic response, and support the overall process. Meditation, mindfulness practice, and loving kindness practice shift old negative habits in the way you view yourself and the world to new, enlivening, and loving ones.

If you would like support on your journey, there is a team of caring, trained people who offer coaching and inspiration, which is the juice that keeps it all flowing and helps you to adjust to the shifts and changes as they occur on your road to a happy and healthy mind, body, and life. In the Resources section, you will find sources for coaching while on the Plan.

If We Are What We Eat, What Does That Make Us?

When the statement "We are what we eat" started to be a buzz many years ago, nutrition was still a budding science. People were intrigued by the idea but had not yet really seen how devastating the results would be to themselves and future generations when they succumbed to mass production and commercialization; packaged foods with all their additives, colorings, and preservatives; and fast food with its addictive flavorings and taste enhancements.

The documentary film *Super Size Me*, the story of Morgan Spurlock, a 32-year-old American man who ate nothing but McDonalds for a month, began a trend. Some people actually began to sit up and take notice of what they were putting in their body and the effect that might have on their health.

Setting himself up well in advance of his little escapade, Morgan had all his vitals checked by several doctors. All of them said he would be surprised at what little change there would be at the completion of this exercise. Instead, it took him more than a full year to recover from the high blood pressure and cholesterol, stifled digestion, constipation, excessive bloating, liver congestion, and 24.5-pound (11 kg) weight gain that he engendered during his one-month experiment. The results, particularly the length of his recovery period, shocked the doctors, and no doubt, Spurlock himself. It also shocked the public, although it was downplayed by the fast-food industry, and his film never got the exposure it deserved. Sadly, it never reached the audience that most needed to hear its message, the low-mid-income North Americans who are most impacted by the deleterious effects of a fast-food diet.

In his book *In Defense of Food*, Michael Pollan discusses the trend toward measuring the nutritional content of the food we buy. Beginning more than fifteen years ago, food manufacturers have been required to include nutritional information on their product packaging. Quoting Marion Nestle, a New York University nutritionist, Pollan notes that the nutritional values on food labels are not an accurate value of what the food provides once it is digested: "The problem with nutrient-by-nutrient nutrition science," Nestle points out, "is that it takes the nutrient out of the context of the food, the food out of the context of the diet, and the diet out of the context of the lifestyle."

We can all rationalize consuming fast food once in while, but once in a while is not the norm. Fast food now exists in every super-market and grocery store. Unaware moms buy fast food daily, giving in to their kids' addictions to colorings, preservatives, and additives; attractive packaging; and superhero marketing techniques. Teenagers and older people are looking for microwaveable ease or freezer-to-plate new-style TV dinners and handheld pizzas, burritos, or whatever else they can find to nuke and eat on the run.

For our "Barbie and Ken" role-model society, the news is that none of this food will deliver that image long-term. It will deliver the same results as those experienced by the young man in *Super Size Me*. We may indeed be turning into human constructs of all the plastics we are ingesting—oil by-products, chemical compounds, and preservatives—but that's where the resemblance to hand-some Ken and perfect Barbie stops short. We're in pretty bad shape. Obesity is at an all-time high, and even though the American public has been aware of it for years, statistics show that in 2009 it was still on the increase.[1] Baffling new autoimmune diseases, cancer, heart disease, and mental illness are increasing at an alarming rate.

Xenoestrogens, herbicides, pesticides, GMOs, food additives, MSG, food colorings, and more all alter our body, our hormones, our mental capacity, our lifespan, our immune function, and our general well-being.

The Omnivore's Dilemma and *In Defense of*

---

[1] Centers for Disease Control and Prevention (CDC), "U.S. Obesity Trends: Trends by State 1985–2009," www.cdc.gov/obesity/data/trends.html.

NOTES

Food, both by Michael Pollan, and *Diet for a New America* and *The Food Revolution* by John Robbins, renegade son of Baskin-Robbins, the ice cream family, are just a few in a long list of books that support clean eating and the obvious resulting good health.

High-Stress, High-Pressure Lifestyle

In addition to being what we eat, our lifestyle has gotten way out of whack. We are not Barbie and Ken in that department either.

If you think that the high-stress, high-pressure lives we lead have no impact on our psyche, emotional nature, and well-being, think again. We see results of our lifestyle around us every day, often up close and personal. A girl has a panic attack at the office when she is unable to meet her production deadline. Our best friend's daughter does caffeine pills to cram for a final and ends up in the hospital with heart palpitations and splitting headaches, needing a spinal tap to recover. Our mothers are on antidepressants or antianxiety meds at seventy. Our kids, and now our forty-year-old girlfriends, are on Ritalin for ADD and ADHD.

Energy: What Makes It and What Takes It!

We don't breathe, and we often don't exercise.[2] In fact, only about sixteen percent of people aged fifteen years and older who live in the United States participated in sports and exercise activities on an average day in recent years.[3] In Canada the statistics are similar.[4] In Australia the average is between twenty-four and twenty-six percent for both men and women.[5] Often, when we do participate, we overexercise,[6] we don't take time to sit down for meals, and we swallow things whole, thinking that food or high-fructose corn syrup with caffeine hits is what gives us energy.

Now, after reading all this, the normal response is to go into mental resistance, total denial, or you could sit down and figure out where you sit in this paradigm of dysfunctionality. Right now you could be one of those people who actually lives life, takes time to shop, has regular family time at meals, enjoys their work, takes time to play with their kids and their spouse—and takes time alone to meditate, breathe, and exercise. Or right now you could be one of those overextended, freaked-out people who push too hard at everything, are compulsive achievers, must be the leader of the pack, have their kids booked into every activity possible, never have a sit-down meal except on vacations, overexercise, are terrified of getting older, and make love

---

[2] A 2009 CDC survey showed that only 35% of adults in the United States engaged in regular leisure-time exercise, and 33% engaged in none at all (www.cdc.gov/nchs/fastats/exercise.htm).

[3] U.S. Bureau of Labor Statistics: Spotlight on Statistics, "Sports and Exercise," May 2008, www.bls.gov/spotlight/2008/sports/pdf/sports_bls_spotlight.pdf.

[4] Statistics Canada, "Study: Participation in Sports," February 2008, www.statcan.gc.ca/daily-quotidien/080207/dq080207b-eng.htm.

[5] Australian Bureau of Statistics, "Participation in Sports and Physical Recreation, Australia, 2005–06," February 14, 2007, www.abs.gov.au/ausstats/abs@.nsf/mediareleasesbytitle/85051A8899BB0446CA2572810077450B?OpenDocument.

[6] CDC data from 2006–2007 showed that one-third of respondent-reported nonfatal, medically attended injury episodes occurred while a person was engaged in leisure activities, including sports (www.cdc.gov/nchs/data/factsheets/factsheet_injury.htm).

to their spouse once a month out of obligation, pleasurable or not.

So how does one find balance?

The *Shorter Oxford English Dictionary* defines energy as "force or vigour of expression," "power, actively and effectively used," and the "latent ability or capacity to produce an effect."

We all know what it means *not* to have energy, but where does it come from, and what takes it away? Is it possible that energy is produced by simply having things working?

When a Maserati is built, it is designed to be sleek, fast, and efficient. It is created from the best materials and made to last. We human beings are designed just like that Maserati, and in a much more complex way, to be sleek, bright-eyed, brilliant, beautiful, and efficient. If that is our design, why are we not this way all the time?

Where does the energy go?

Stress

The word *stress* gets a bad rap. Stress is the pressure that holds things together and the force that makes things work, like a kind of universal glue. However, when stress is extreme, imbalances occur and problems arise. Too much stress causes dysfunction, which, in turn, creates *distress*.

Richard Gerber, MD, wrote in his book *Vibrational Medicine: The #1 Handbook of Subtle-Energy Therapies*, "A certain amount of stress is functional to maintaining optimal health. Hans Selye, the pioneering stress researcher, referred to this optimal level of stress as eu-

stress. If this level of stress is exceeded, causing dysfunction in the system, the individual experiences distress." As Selye explained, a certain amount of stress is necessary, but as usual in our Western society, we tend to think that if a little is good, a lot is better; well, in this case, this is not so at all. Overstress, or distress, drains energy.

Body systems that are working inefficiently also drain energy. For example, if our digestive system is impaired, we experience problems such as gas, bloating, reflux, heartburn, high blood sugar, and low blood sugar. When elimination doesn't work smoothly, constipation or diarrhea result and we don't absorb nutrients properly. This puts stress on other systems and we can become dehydrated, our lymphatic system can become congested, and we feel exhausted.

Negative emotions such as worry, anger, or being upset drain energy. We have all experienced exhaustion when worry takes over or felt debilitated by anger or losing our temper. Positive emotions can also drain energy if indulged in to the extreme.

Lack of sleep drains energy. We need sleep to restore our energy, and when our body is running on empty, we are in danger of hormonal, digestive, and emotional imbalance. Exhaustion breeds more exhaustion. In our day-to-day working world, adrenal fatigue is running rampant, so constant tiredness is considered normal.

Lack of oxygen takes energy. We seldom breathe deeply; in fact, we are a society (especially in North America, the UK, Western

Europe, and Australia) that is known to be chest breathers. Unlike people who, like babies, consciously breathe into their abdomen well into adulthood, such as meditators, martial artists, and yoga practitioners, we are oxygen-deprived. This condition makes all our body systems less efficient. Oxygen is essential to convert our food into energy, and our cells must be properly oxygenated in order to function; cells deprived of oxygen will die. Cells need to be properly oxygenated for serotonin levels to be balanced, for proper hormone production, and for all body functions, including the peristaltic wave that controls elimination.

Lack of minerals drains energy. Distress depletes essential trace minerals. Minerals are found in every body tissue and fluid, and they are essential for many body functions, including nerve transmission, muscle contraction, tissue structure, blood formation, acid-alkaline (electrolyte) balance, and energy production. Ensuring the body has a balanced supply of minerals can help combat the effects of stress. In his book *Salt: Your Way to Health*, David Brown-

stein, MD, writes, "Unrefined salt, containing over 80 minerals, is the perfect source of salt for the body. It provides a proper balance of nutrients that the body can use." In Chapter Six, "Coaxing Metabolism," you will learn more about refined versus unrefined sea salt.

Lack of hydration drains energy. The body cannot survive without air and water; they are essential. We can do without food for weeks, but water is essential to all body functions. In his book *Your Body's Many Cries for Water*, Dr. F. Batmanghelidj writes, "Water is the primary nutrient in the body. Water not only generates energy, it carries nutrients to all the tissues of the body." Water is nature's filtration system, so hydration is necessary for detoxifying the cells. Without detoxification, acidosis ensues and conditions such as cancer, autoimmune disorders, arthritis, and premature aging occur. Rather than just water, alkaline water is a much better choice because it neutralizes acidity and detoxifies the body naturally.

Lack of exercise drains energy. Now *that* is an interesting comment! Energy is needed to exercise, but lack of exercise drains en-

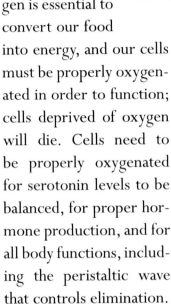

I am now *completely* prescription-*free*, and very proud of it. I have learned much about loving myself and making myself a priority so that I can be the healthy leader God made me to be, and able to share this incredible path to wellness with others.
— *Lisa D., Mother and Wife Crestwood, Kentucky*

ergy. When your body stops exercising, toxins build up in your lymphatic system, your digestive system becomes sluggish and you don't assimilate nutrients or eliminate wastes efficiently, your sleep suffers, and your mental function becomes fuzzy. When you don't move, things get stuck, and when things get stuck, you lose energy.

Extra weight drains energy. If you have ever done a therapy workshop for weight loss, the therapist may have you carry around a 5-pound (2.5 kg) package of flour for a day. If you have never done it, try it out and see how much energy it takes to carry it and how much it gets in your way.

So now that we know some of the things that deplete energy …

What Creates Energy?

The converse of course: systems that work. That cared-for, recently tuned-up Maserati that has a tank full of good, clean, no-additive fuel runs fast, cleanly, and without a hitch. What a joy it is to experience riding in a clean-running, well-lubricated, fully functional machine. You can drive quickly, effortlessly, and without having to pay attention to anything else but the pure fun of a smooth ride—at any speed you wish.

It is the same with our body. When we get sufficient oxygen, pure water, exercise, good clean food, sleep, minerals—and have a structured lifestyle, a good attitude, self-confidence, and love—we feel great. We run like the cared-for Maserati!

So we need more than good food, but how do we get what we need? How do we find the fountain of energy? What is a new lifestyle versus a diet?

NOTES

Habits

Autobiography in Five Short Chapters

Chapter One
I walk down the street.
There is deep hole in the sidewalk.
I fall in.
I am lost ... I am helpless.
It isn't my fault.
It takes forever to find a way out.

Chapter Two
I walk down the same street.
There is deep hole in the sidewalk.
I pretend I don't see it.
I fall in again.
I can't believe I am in this same place.
But it isn't my fault.
It still takes a long time to get out.

Chapter Three
I walk down the same street.
There is deep hole in the sidewalk.
I see it is there.
I still fall in ... it is a habit ... but,
my eyes are open.
I know where I am.
It is *my* fault.
I get out immediately.

Chapter Four
I walk down the same street.
There is a deep hole in the sidewalk.
I walk around it.

Chapter Five
I walk down another street.
— Portia Nelson, *There's a Hole in My
Sidewalk: The Romance of Self-Discovery*

Discipline is a word that often gives us trouble. It looks like sacrifice, loss of freedom, domination, and rigidity. The truth is, we all have our ingrained habits, and whether they're beneficial or harmful they require diligence and discipline. You may not see it that way—especially when it comes to the discipline of laziness. In his book *Mindfulness in Plain English*, Bhante Henepola Gunaratana captures so well my feelings on this topic:

> "Discipline" is a difficult word for most of us. It conjures up images of somebody standing over you with a stick, telling you that you're wrong. But self-discipline is different. It's the skill of seeing through the hollow shouting of your own impulses and piercing their secret. They have no power over you. It's all a show, a deception. Your urges scream and bluster at you; they cajole; they coax; they threaten; but they really carry no stick at all. You give in to them out of habit. You give in because you never really bother to look beyond the threat. It is all empty back there. There is only one way to learn this lesson, though. The words on this page won't do it. But look within and watch the stuff coming up—restlessness, anxiety, impatience, pain—just watch it come up and don't get involved. Much to your surprise, it will simply go away. It rises, it passes away. As simple as that. There is another word for self-discipline. It is patience.

Discipline and patience move us toward developing diligence. That diligence gives one a sense of accomplishment and strength of character that can be relied on, at all times, but especially in times of duress or when we are tempted to give in to old habits that die hard. "Do no harm" is one of the main constructs of the principle of discipline in Eastern philosophy. This principle begins with the application of doing no harm to ourselves. Courage is what eventually develops, courage to continue, to persevere and find kindness toward ourselves and others as a way of life.

It takes three weeks or twenty-one days to make or break a habit. The people who run the detox treatment centers will tell you that's why most of their programs are for six weeks: three weeks to break the cycle and three weeks to establish a new one.

Real Food

In his book *In Defense of Food*, Michael Pollan refers to "real food." His claim is that we have become a nation of nutritionally challenged individuals, having to look at package labels to determine the protein, carbohydrate, sugar, sodium, and energy content of food. Real food has no such packaging. Produce is fresh, alive, unfrozen, untreated, and vibrant; poultry, meat, and eggs are fresh. If there is a way for you to get organic or pasture-raised, free-range chicken, beef, and lamb, and organic, or at least locally grown, pesticide- and herbicide-free produce, that is ideal. Fish should be wild-caught, not farm-raised. Chemicals are not nutritious. Biodynamic farming, based on Rudolph Steiner's principles, is growing throughout the Western world. Foxhollow Farm in Crestwood, Kentucky, owned by Janie Newton, is just one example of how this style of farming is showing up in our culture. The philosophy is one of working in harmony with nature, where the earth is regarded as a living being. Our bodies are alive, and they survive best on live food, freshly prepared, with its vibrancy still intact.

The current sustainability culture growing wildly in the United States and Canada focuses on these values. Hopefully, the movement will catch on and people will again begin to garden, shop at local farmers' markets, and get their meat, fish, and produce locally—clean and fresh.

Real Water

My father was a water-well driller. He was always ahead of his time and had the most modern equipment in the world. Dad always predicted the level of water pollution that would occur within our lifetime. He spoke of bottled water and lakes where no one could swim safely, of fish dying, of pollution, and of the poisoning of our waterways and farmlands. He predicted the takeover in agriculture by the chemical producers. The small town where I grew up fell right into line with many of his predictions. The main source of employment was a Uniroyal chemical plant, or the Naugatuck Chemical Company, as it was called when I was growing up in Ontario, Canada.

In the sixties and seventies, the local waterways were the source of tumor-laden fish; kids who swam in the Canagagigue Creek in Elmira often became ill, and the development of sepsis in small cuts and wounds was considered normal. The level of mental

NOTES

retardation in the area was also considered normal. It was thought to be high because of the closed-community nature of the local Mennonites and Amish, but I often wonder if there was more to it than that. Eventually, the company was prosecuted for damage to the environment and to the town's water source. People sued for damages when the water and the soil next to the river in the surrounding farmland were shown to be toxic.

Many cities are now claiming that their tap water is safe to drink. *Safe* has many interpretations, as does the word *natural*, which is bandied around and applied to all kinds of very unnatural substances. Marketing is a wonderful thing, but people are naive. Local water, wherever you are, is probably not "safe" to drink. Even if it is safe, it may not be the best source of drinking water. One of the best oncologists I know of, when seeing patients for the first time, immediately takes them off tap water and puts them on reverse-osmosis, oxygen-enriched, alkaline water. If the medical community is savvy enough to do this, perhaps "safe" is not the word we should be using for tap water. Water also needs to be alive. It needs to have magnetic resonance. It needs to be an able filter for the body, providing the hydration it needs to function optimally. In addition, the chemicals added to water, including fluoride (which has a debilitating effect on thyroid function), as well as the water purification processes, make water less available for assimilation by the body.

As it is processed, cleaned, and put out through long miles of pipeline to supply the public, water loses its natural magnetic energy. Pipes and processing reduce its ability to oxygenate. Water is nature's and the body's most effective filtration system, and it is important to have real, live, activated water, as much as you need, daily. Each person requires a slightly different volume of water, but you should never become thirsty, because then you have already passed "the need for hydration" mark.

Six ounces (180 mL) of water each hour is roughly what your body can assimilate, unless you are doing heavy exercise or are exposed to excessive heat or cold. Under those conditions you need more. Many people have been brainwashed into gulping down great volumes of water all at once, and then going for hours with no other hydration. This heightens kidney and bladder stress. Small sips of water over a longer time period is a much more effective plan, and this strategy is even more efficient if you have fluid retention. The body will stop holding fluid if you keep the supply of fresh, oxygenated, alkaline water readily available. Keep a toxin-free plastic or glass bottle of fresh water around wherever you are, or even better, carry it with you. And it is water that you need, not just fluid, so coffee, juice, tea (except herbal), and soda don't count.

It is wisest to consume alkaline water because it alkalizes the body and helps prevent acidic conditions, which can have a negative effect on many organs. Acidity and inflammation, its cousin, are contributing factors in the epidemic increase in chronic disease.

If you do not have a source of alkaline water through a purification process or straight from the earth, then add trace minerals to make it more alkaline. Adding a pinch of unprocessed sea salt or sea minerals, or a dash of apple cider vinegar, will spice it up if you are not a person who enjoys drinking water. You will find that alkalized water is silky and feels wonderful going down the throat.

Breath Is Life

Breath

Are you looking for me? I am in the next
    seat.
My shoulder is against yours.

You will not find me in the stupas, not in
    Indian shrine rooms,
nor in synagogues, nor in cathedrals:
not in masses, nor kirtans, not in legs
    winding around your own neck,
nor in eating nothing but vegetables.
When you really look for me, you will see
    me instantly—
you will find me in the tiniest house of time.
Kabir says: Student, tell me what is God?
He is the breath inside the breath.
    — Kabir (1440–1518), Indian Poet-Saint
        (as translated by Robert Bly)

In 2007 I did a three-day retreat for participants in the Plan (then called the Swissplan)

NOTES

at Foxhollow, a beautiful retreat center close to Louisville, Kentucky (now a working farm dedicated to becoming completely organic and biodynamic). Each morning we did a series of breathwork exercises. Part of the introduction involved watching a DVD called *Nooma: Breathe 14* by Rob Bell, a young, innovative pastor from Minnesota (please see the Resources section). Although it was just a short fourteen-minute DVD, when we watched it and heard Bell speak of the spiritual nature of breath, we all became truly inspired. He quoted experts, saying, "Ninety-nine percent of our energy should come from our breath, and they say that most of us access between ten and twenty percent of that energy."

As the weekend progressed, I began to see the color come into people's faces, a spring show up in their step, and a glimmer and twinkle appear in their eyes. The participants noticed that their digestive pattern had changed; they felt happier and more positive, energized, and better in general. They were breathing. There are many parts to the Plan that bring these changes to bear, but one of the first to produce an obvious effect on all levels is breathing.

When I began to develop this particular type of breathing regimen, I was in a long-term (three-year) focused practice retreat with Sogyal Rinpoche, a Tibetan teacher with whom I study. Another Tibetan teacher had taught me the basics of breathing many years before.

One of the younger Tibetans, another Rinpoche (a Tibetan term meaning "precious teacher") had been invited to speak to the participants. Tsognyi Rinpoche was an expert in the *lung* (pronounced *loong*) breathing technique. Several months later, he came to Louisville to offer a short retreat and to give his personal retreat participants detailed instructions with regard to breath. I attended that retreat. I now attempt to offer a simplified version of this breathing technique and provide this particular breathing style, together with the attitude that accompanies it to, hopefully, ease the stress people experience mentally and emotionally from locked-up wind (or lung) energy.

The link between breath and the soul is recognized in many cultures throughout the world. In Hebrew, the word *ruah* means "spirit," "breath," or "wind." In Tibetan, the word *lung* has a similar reference and is employed in Tibetan medicine to describe a necessary element for balance and well-being of the body, mind, and spirit, the lack of which results in disease. It involves not only breath but also cognitive and emotional energetic pathways and their resultant flow through the body.

The Chinese considered the breath so vital that the symbol for it in the Chinese characters of writing is the same as that for rice, the staff of life for the Chinese people. The word is *chi*. To avoid confusion with the same word used in energy medicine, *chi* of breath was referred to as *inner chi*.

The Romans coined the Latin word *respiritus* for breath. *Re* means "return to" and *spiritus* is the word for "spirit." In everyday

English, "respire" just means "to breathe," but in its Latin origin, it means "return to spirit." "Expire" is the word for "breathing out," but also means "to die," or a disconnection of spirit from body.

Throughout millennia, breath has been a part of all healing structures concerned with well-being—the settling of mind, increasing blood flow, and improving the functionality of the body's organs. This is so for all cultures except ours. Perhaps it is because we are such a mix of cultures that some of the really valuable rituals, knowledge, and practices have become lost in our smorgasbord of Western reality, or maybe it is just stress.

The only way that we seem to get breath is to run; work out; or work ourselves into a cardio frenzy in a sweaty, loud-music environment that is anything but inspiring. All of these methods involve force rather than choice and a lack of sensitivity to the breath and its profound effects. Even the styles of yoga adapted to our Western taste are often strenuous; ashtanga yoga and hot yoga demand stamina and strength, fulfilling our need for stimulation and push. However, because breath is an integral component of all yoga, the original yoga styles work more with the gentler aspects of breath. I have trouble denying the advantages of combining breath, sweat, and focus, since I taught hot yoga and still go to classes whenever I can, but the slower, gentler methods are often what we as a culture need more.

An Ancient Point of Reference

The Taoist, Tibetan, and Ayurvedic traditions of medicine rely on the breath as the source of evenness, not only on a physical level but also emotionally, mentally, and spiritually. In

NOTES

the Tibetan tradition, it is said that the breath is the horse and the mind is the rider, the point being that we must tame the horse and also the rider. From the point of view of these Eastern medicine practices, balance is found with breath, creating a condition in the body and mind less conducive to disease and distress.

Disease states develop differently in Eastern and Western cultures, although the East is quickly adopting our habits and, as a result, developing our diseases as well.

Cognitive and Emotional Congestion

On reflection, you may notice that many Western diseases are centered in the head. Blockages occur frequently in the head because Westerners are cognitively and intellectually focused, and therefore well developed in the head. Also, our most common problem is that we think too much. The Tibetan medicine term *lung* (pronounced *loong*), or "wind," affects patterns of energy and movement in the body, as well as the mind and nervous system.

The other area of congestion with regard to breath, or more accurately, *lung*, is the solar plexus (just below the breast bone). Tibetan medicine says that congestion in the solar plexus is a result of being emotionally underdeveloped. In our culture, we lean toward volatility and passion, in both a negative and a positive sense. We are often flighty and not in control of our emotions. This does not apply to every individual, of course, but most of us would agree that we seldom breathe into the solar plexus unless under physical duress.

We are highly emotional beings, and much of our emotional expression is uncontrolled. Anger, lust, fear, depression, and anxiety are commonplace emotions for many people. If we are not indulging these emotions as encouraged by our media and fast-paced lives, we

> **I am calmer, not so anxious. I sleep, as my mother used to say, 'Like a brick.' My hormones are balanced. I eliminate each time I eat. The puffiness is all gone, my hands and feet don't swell on a long trip, and I am smaller and thinner. Finding an eating pattern that works is nothing short of life-altering and life-lengthening. My quality of life is back. I have energy and the *joie de vivre* each of God's creatures should have.**
>
> — *Eunice R., National VP, Arbonne Crestwood, Kentucky*

16

often suppress them according to our judgment of what is right and wrong.

Diseases and conditions regarding congestion in the head have increased dramatically in the last twenty years, including brain tumors, Alzheimer's, Parkinson's, aneurysms, psychoses, anxiety, and depression.

In the solar plexus and thoracic area of the body, conditions that are increasing—in some cases to epidemic proportions—are panic attacks, asthma, digestive conditions, breast cancer, lung cancer, heart disease, lymphatic cancers, hepatitis, liver cancer, and pancreatic dysfunctions, including cancer and diabetes.

In changing our habitual patterns of breathing, which contribute to congestion in these two areas specifically, perhaps we can shift the propensity for these disease states in our own body and change some emotional leanings as well.

Inspiration: Breath Brings Life

When trying to overcome extreme anxiousness and depression, it is important to learn the techniques of correct breathing. Most people living with high levels of anxiety and/or stressful lifestyles tend to breathe from the chest rather than the abdomen. Shallow breathing disrupts the balance of oxygen and carbon dioxide necessary for a relaxed state. Shallow breathing actually perpetuates the symptoms of anxiety.

The Wave

In addition to reducing anxiety and depression, breathing into your belly and holding it there for a short count brings balance to brain chemistry and hormones. Breathing in this way also helps "the wave"—the peristaltic movement that assists the digestive process of ingestion, appropriation, assimilation, and

NOTES

elimination. Low-belly (abdominal) breathing helps to eliminate fat in the belly area. This type of belly fat is generated by insulin resistance and the accumulation of estrogen-retaining fat in both men and women. In addition, at times of stress the adrenal hormone cortisol causes fat to be deposited in the abdomen. Released by the adrenal glands, cortisol can cause major imbalances in blood sugar levels and a decrease in bone density and pain response. Deep breathing reduces stress, and thus an overproduction of cortisol.

The Natural Pattern of Breath

Deep, diaphragmatic breathing is an efficient way to assist the body in reducing anxiety, depression, and the effects of stress. We automatically breathe this way when we are born and continue breathing this way as young children. If you watch children sleeping, you will see their belly rise and fall with each breath.

This style of taking in breath uses the diaphragm muscle, the strong dome-shaped muscle located under our ribs and above our stomach. When we breathe in, we push the muscle down, and our lower belly (abdomen) moves out. When we breathe out, the diaphragmatic muscle moves back to resting position and our belly moves back in.

During infancy and early childhood, we breathe naturally from the diaphragm. As we grow older, most of us change from our original pattern of breathing and start breathing from our chest. At this stage, we are no longer breathing naturally. This can be the result of a number of factors, such as poor posture, too much time spent in a seated po-

sition, or the depression posture of a caved-in chest and slumped shoulders. Other reasons for this unnatural form of breathing can be the tendency to focus energy in the head by thinking and worrying, and then taking short breaths when under duress.

Lack of physical exercise, current fashions, and the pressure on women and men to have flat stomachs (muffin-tops over the jeans and beer bellies are not cool) add to the problem. Holding in your stomach for fashion is good for the muscles and the look, but not for healthy breathing. A soft belly is not as fashionable, but it is much easier to breathe into. Most shallow or chest breathing is associated with some form of stress or distress, a type of holding, either physical, emotional, or both.

The Method

To become aware of your breathing, place one hand on your upper chest and one on your belly, four fingers below your navel. You need to do this only at the beginning to get a sense of where the breath goes and to give it focus. Breathe in through your nose, taking in an even stream of air as though you were breathing through a straw. As you breathe in, let your tongue rise to the roof of your mouth and bring the air down into your belly. Let your stomach swell out and expand. (You may have to undo your jeans to do this.)

As you breathe out, let your stomach come back gently. Try to get a steady rhythm going, taking the same depth of breath each time. Your mouth should be softly closed, with your lips and jaws relaxed, or slightly open if your jaws clench with closing. The hand on your chest should have little or no movement out, as there should be only a slight expansion to the sides and lower part of your chest. Take the same depth of breath each time you breathe in, breathing slowly, steadily, and deeply into your belly.

The Next Step

When you begin to feel comfortable with this technique, try to slow your breathing rate down by putting in a short pause after you have breathed in and before you breathe out again. Initially it may feel as though you are not getting enough air, but with regular practice this slower breathing rate will soon start to feel comfortable. The next step is to allow the breath to be evenly taken in and allow your belly to extend outward. Hold the breath with your belly extended for several seconds before breathing out. A good starting point seems to be a very slow count of six, slowing it down even more as you become more comfortable.

The long-term objective is to breathe most of the time with your belly and not your chest, aiming for about six to eight breaths per minute. This will require holding the breath in your lower belly each time for as much as fifteen to twenty counts—the longer, the better. This is a slow, relaxed process; it shouldn't take effort. Increase the counts as you feel you are able.

NOTES

The Mind Effect

Focusing on the in and out rhythm of the breath has a meditative effect, and developing this rhythm will prevent other thoughts from entering your mind. If you become aware of other thoughts, just notice them as they show up and let them go. Bring your attention back to the breath; breathe in, belly out, pause, hold, breathe out, belly in; breathe in, belly out, pause, hold, breathe out, belly in.

Keeping the *lung* energy, which travels down from the head, through the solar plexus, and down below the navel, with at least fifteen percent in the belly, and then back up again is something to work toward. Each of us has a propensity to tighten up and hold in one area or the other—head or solar plexus— wherever we get a little more stuck when stressed. When stress is high, we often trap the *lung* energy in both areas. While doing the breathwork, hold an intention for the *lung* energy to move down into the belly with the breath.

When to Do It and the Result

If you practice this technique for ten minutes twice a day, and for a shorter time whenever you become aware of the constriction of your breath—when you are restless, anxious, fearful, or depressed—you will begin to strengthen the responsiveness to breath and find more ease in extending your abdomen. You will experience relaxation and mind clarity right away. Developing this skill will leave you with a nice, relaxed feeling of ease, a clear head, and a sense of calm. You will be very capable of concentrating and focusing.

Breathing this way in the morning and taking a few moments to do it throughout the day will help you shift toward a state of mind less dominated by thinking and emotion.

This does not have to be a dramatic exercise; you can do it in the car or even in a business meeting. You might have to make it a little more outwardly obvious and dramatic at first to get your body accustomed to the practice, but then drop the drama and just integrate it into your normal everyday way of being.

Deepening the Skill

Any *lung* energy, breath, and focus trapped in the head, the solar plexus, or the heart area, is often what causes us to feel disoriented, fearful, and in a state of panic. In the West this feeling is becoming commonplace and accepted as normal, which is not the case at all. If you wish to feel peaceful and at ease, the *lung* must be moved back down to its place of origin four fingers below the navel. In order to remain calm consistently, fifteen to twenty percent of the breath should remain in this center. That's the goal.

The first step in the second stage, deepening the skill, is to scan your body with your mind and discover where your trapped *lung* sits. It may be in your head, your throat, your chest, heart area, or your solar plexus. If you often have headaches and worry, the *lung* might be trapped in the head. If you withhold your self-expression and suppress your opinions, you may hold it in your throat. If you have a tendency to panic attacks or are overly responsible, you might hold *lung* energy in your heart area. If you are overly emotional or fearful and often feel attacked, you may hold it in your solar plexus. You get the idea? It also may drift from one area to another. Just look and see where it is at the time you are doing this exercise and work with it.

The breathing technique, the method described in the first exercise, is an important precursor to the intention to return the *lung* to its home below the navel. The only difference in this second skill is that the breath, once taken in, is then held for as long as you can. Masters can hold the breath for thirty seconds. This is a focus to aim for, since at the beginning you will not be able to do this without strain and should not even try. As you begin to do this exercise, hold the breath as long as you are able to without strain. As I said before, a slow count of six is a good start.

Your mouth in this case is closed, or very slightly open. Your chin is tucked, your eyes can be open or closed, and your tongue is on the roof of your mouth. Breath is drawn in through your nose, slowly and in a paced, relaxed fashion. Your belly is extended and your pelvic area expands, whereas your chest remains relaxed, as does your solar plexus. If you cannot manage this at the beginning of the work, just "fake-it-till-you-make-it"; in other words, imagine it, visualize it in your mind, and try to emulate it in your physical expression until your body starts to cooperate. Remember to maintain your intention and to gently bring the *lung* energy down. It also helps to watch yourself in the mirror with that intent, standing sideways, and observing your body as it goes through the motions. Breathe in, belly fills up; hold, count, and breathe out, belly goes in.

NOTES

Chew Your Way through It

Chewing is a part of the digestive process that somehow has been forgotten. A third of our digestive power occurs in the mouth. In fact, digestion begins with the enzymes released by our mouth as we chew. Sitting down at the table with the place set with a plate, knife, and fork, and drinking little while eating, except for sips of water, beer, or wine, complete the ritual of eating.

So how does it all work and why is chewing so important?

The salivary glands produce an enzyme called *amylase* that breaks down simple starches in our foods. The longer we chew, the more the food we eat is broken down and, therefore, the more food particles are bathed in amylase, which prepares it for the next stage of digestion in the stomach. As a result, the more thoroughly we chew our food, the more efficiently we digest it.

Chewing every bite of food at least thirty times sets up the following reactions:

- Chewing sends messages to your stomach about the nature and amount of food that is about to be digested. If your stomach is alerted ahead of time about the food that is coming, it can prepare the right amount of stomach acid.
- According to university studies, chewing stimulates the endocrine system, keeping your hormones in balance for a happier, younger-looking you.
- The parotid glands just under your cheekbones release a cell-rejuvenating substance as you chew.

- The more you chew, the more oxygen is sent to your brain. Munching is magnificent for the memory.

Starting the digestive process in this way stimulates the entire digestive response, resulting in a smoother transition, better assimilation, and less stress on the organs, especially the stomach, pancreas, liver, and small intestine. More energy is then available to you.

In addition to all of these wonderful reasons, mindfully taking time for yourself to sit and chew when you eat is an important way to refocus and center yourself. Some clients have said they have often eaten an extra meal when they rushed because they had trouble remembering if they had eaten that meal previously. Eating on the run, they were simply too preoccupied to notice. For a European, this would be inconceivable and heartbreaking, disloyal to the gustatory tradition. Most people who begin to chew their food well immediately reduce or eliminate heartburn, reflux, gas, and bloating. I have seen this transformation occur so often with my clients who are on medication for reflux; within a few days of breathing and chewing, they no longer need their medication.

Sitting down to eat with a knife and fork (it can be plastic or you can carry your own cutlery with you if you are not at home) is important. Focusing on chewing thirty times with each bite and putting utensils down between bites makes a difference. Focusing on chewing, not a television, computer, or newspaper, is best. It is not always going to be possible, but hold an intention to bring more order and structure into your life with the goal of sitting down at a dining room table, if possible, with a nice place setting (place mat or tablecloth, plates, napkin, knife, fork, spoon, glass, and cup). Do this as often as possible and you will start to see the difference.

Many of you will actually find this ritual of eating a foreign experience. A few of you will have never done this before except on special occasions. Why not try it? Make sitting down to eat a daily ritual, and you might like it. It will make you feel special, like royalty; and when you treat yourself like royalty you will feel like royalty. Can't be bad, right?

NOTES

Cycled Patterns of Living

CHAPTER THREE

The Importance of Structure and Ritual

For much of our past, humans have been agrarian, agriculturists, farmers. For thousands of years we followed the same patterns. As habit and ritual tamed our bodies and psyches, our biological clocks developed around this model as well.

Our ancestors lived with Nature and followed her commands. Every morning they rose with the sun, and before heading out to work in the fields, broke their fast (that's how the word "breakfast" came into being). They stopped at midday, when the sun was high, and the family got together in the fields for the main meal of the day. They ate together, watched the children play, and then had a nap to let the meal digest, thus avoiding work under the hot midday sun. After the siesta, work in the fields continued until dusk, when they returned home for a light dinner before sunset, and then to bed. How civilized!

Humanity was not automated then, nor did we have electricity to create a false sense of day and night. We also did not have —

- the imposed external time demands of work hours that are not connected to natural cycles of time;
- excessive social agendas carrying us far into electrically lit evenings;
- stress that compels us to eat whenever we are even slightly hungry;
- a lack of ritual around food (e.g., eating

from containers while standing up, instead of sitting down to a relaxing meal, and grazing);

- the habit of bolting our food (only to return to what seems more important—whatever was interrupted by our craving, hunger, and justification to eat);

- the urge to eat at random, unstructured times out of boredom, emotional suppression, or distraction; and

- advertisers bombarding us with visual stimulation to eat what we see on TV or on billboards, often from the familiar fast-food outlets, and the timing is often right around mealtime.

What Happened?

In addition to eating at odd times, a habit we've developed over the past fifty years as our lives have become more automated and fast-paced, we eat foods that aren't real. We devour huge amounts of fast food and packaged food with ingredients that make us crave more of these very foods. No wonder overeating is so common. The food we eat is filled with stimulants and addictive substances.

Caffeine, sugar, sugar substitutes, sodium, MSG, preservatives, food coloring, and other additives all create a false need for continually eating them, as they often have an addictive or stimulating quality—sometimes both. Since mealtimes have disappeared, we no longer give any consideration to the timing of our food intake. Our food packaging is organized in such a way that many small meals seem better than eating a lot at a time. That, too, is a deceptive form of marketing. Along with popular fad diets, even the natural-food and personal-training industries endorse and promote "grazing." Being busy, stressed, and tired, we've become lazy about food preparation, so we've willingly bought right into the grazing craze. Don't misunderstand me, there are some people for whom the grazing patterns seem to work, but I have found that, even with them, the three-meals-a-day regimen helps regulate metabolic response and makes them more settled.

When Do Our Organs Get to Rest?

All of this has shot our body's intricate systems into a state of overuse, confusion, and havoc. The systems we feed by taking nutrition in any form other than real food—pills, powders, or packaged items—are among those badly affected by our modern lifestyle. We do not respect the natural cycles of our body, nor do we listen to what it really needs. Of all the abuses of our modern society, none is as profound as what we do to our own body and its organs and systems with what is being substituted for food.

I host a monthly day of free drop-in consultation clinics as part of my community service. These are run by Rainbow Blossom Natural Foods, a small chain of natural-food stores in Louisville, Kentucky. On the first Monday of every month, people line up for fifteen-minute sessions. Most are curious about an alternative take on their illness. It is wise on their part, since many suffer from chronic ill health, many due to prescription drug abuse, a sedentary lifestyle, and nutritional deficiencies.

What continues to shock me is that so many people without a surplus of available cash can be brainwashed by newspapers and other media and become financially strapped from ingesting drugs, supplements, powders, and pills instead of food. They are literally starving themselves eating junk food, frozen dinners, corn syrup–laden drinks, and sweet snacks, assuming the drugs and supplements will make up the difference. Under these conditions, their body must work even harder, and ultimately becomes an acidic, inflammation-producing machine. Please don't get me wrong here, I could not do the work I do with people without supplements. The misunderstanding by the public is that pills will take the place of real food.

Addicted to Stimulation

Because our eating and assimilation of real food has become so dysfunctional, the resulting lack of energy leads us to develop a distorted sense of need for stimulants. The ups and downs of overstimulation and undernourishment create a highly volatile, and stressed, internal environment. Our body struggles to maintain balance and has to juggle too many balls to allow the digestive and energy-producing processes to work efficiently.

Like a badly maintained car that wears down quickly, we do not fare well with such neglect. Weak spots, either congenital (inherited) or chronic (the result of previous breakdown), or from accumulated wear and tear, become even weaker. The immune system lacks the resilient strength to respond; it, too, is weakened by the lack of proper assimilation combined with the stress factors in our daily lives. In spite of all the medications and surgeries available to us, we are fast becom-

NOTES

ing less healthy than humans have been in the history of humanity. We may statistically be living longer, but our quality of life is questionable. People seldom die of natural causes nowadays, but rather of some state of disease that often begins in middle age and frequently stems from overstimulation and undernourishment.

Running with Your Body Clock

While I was writing this book in rural France, my daily rituals were simple: I arose before dawn, walked, meditated, cared for the early-morning needs of the animals, ate breakfast in silence, wrote, went to the garden for fresh sun-warmed tomatoes, ate lunch under the trees, *j'ai fait la sieste*, exercised the horses, ate dinner, and went to bed. Each day had the same rhythm. There was softness to that rhythm—safety. Insight and inspiration to write came easily, without effort.

Structures in time are like structures of buildings; they offer space and refuge. The environment of the dramatically beautiful yet simple French countryside offered space, and the rhythm (once I surrendered to it) was heavenly, allowing me to let go with the flow of time and nature.

I spent my summers as a young girl on my grandmother's farm. I really looked forward to those times. Days were always the same. We rose at seven, washed our faces, made our beds, and went downstairs for hot cereal and fruit with toast. We always ate lunch at noon and dinner at six. We took long, leisurely walks to Lake Huron, a few miles away, spent most of the day there, and picked berries along the side of the road in the summer sun as we sauntered back in the late afternoon. We spent time picking sour cherries from the big old cherry tree, shaking the apple tree so the ripe ones would fall, digging for new potatoes, and going to the neighbor's to gather fresh eggs and wonderful milk with cream settled on the top. Bedtime was usually between nine and ten, close to sundown in the Ontario summertime. Grandma allowed no snacks because "you will spoil your dinner," and no sweets except on special occasions, because "you don't want cavities when you go to the dentist." It was a simple, safe, sweet, and trustworthy life, connected with the cycles of nature and the body. Sound sleep and rosy cheeks were guaranteed. We felt alive!

Most action patterns in nature are associated with cycles of time, following the principle of circadian rhythms: cycles of waking, sleeping, activity, and eating. All animals listen to these cycles and act with them, and so did human beings until relatively recently, when we started making up our own clock.

Circadian rhythms and biological clocks are nature's way. It's a pattern that feels stable and grounded because it is in tune with the body's cycles of digestion and the appropriate times of day for all functions. There is an internal balancing that goes on when people follow this natural cycle: The body is at ease, hormones are balanced, digestion is optimal, energy is high, and mental faculties are at their peak. Inner peace is almost always the result.

The Illusion of Day and Night

The pineal gland is a tiny endocrine gland located near the middle of the brain that affects the modulation of the patterns of sleep and awake times. It controls the production and release of the hormone melatonin. The pineal gland is one of the organs affected in a profoundly negative way by our current lifestyle

Days now are falsely extended. Electricity enables us to stay up late into the dark night, and we often get up after sunrise. Because we are out of sync with natural rhythms, many of us have no real appetite for breakfast. Then, due to the frenetic pace of the day, we often have little or no time for lunch, so we either grab something on the run, or miss the meal altogether. We eat a late and leisurely dinner, since it is the only time we have to relax. Think about it: We are so busy we use our only downtime for eating. None of this is in sync with nature's cycle for digestion, nor does it support the digestion and assimilation our body needs to generate more energy—the ultimate purpose of eating. When we are young, the body is forgiving—not so as we age, when energy declines.

The agrarian model still exists in some places around the globe (France is one of those places), and in places where there are no food shortages, the health of the people is better than ours. In the Western world, parts of France, Spain, Italy, and some places in South America still follow that agricultural model. Statistically, those cultures do much better than North American and British cultures (including the colonies) with regard to wellness, and a good part of that comes from their lifestyle priorities and how and what they eat.

The following schedule is the natural timing dictated by nature. It has been established

NOTES

as the healthiest times for you to eat, be active, and sleep, according to the cycles of your body and its connection with the natural rhythms of nature. And as my teacher always told me, every hour you sleep before midnight gives you double the quality of rest.

Breakfast: between 4 and 8 a.m.
Lunch: between 11 a.m. and 1:30 p.m.
Dinner: between 5 and 6:30 or 7 p.m.
Bedtime: 10 p.m.

Cycles of Digestion

The body has predetermined processes of action. The cycles of digestion are just one of the cycles of creation and action that exist in the body's system for supporting itself. Another is reproduction, and we all know it takes nine months of gestation for a baby to develop. In the same way, it takes a year to totally renovate your digestive system. Putting the habits into place that support change is a vital part of the Plan and its principles.

Renewal

Every year your body renews itself on the cellular level, and every seven years you are actually a completely new person. Taking advantage of this wonder of nature is an opportunity you don't want to miss. Consider that you could actually drop years by simply changing a few things in your daily activities, including what you eat and when. Now this is what I call awesome renovation!

The cycles of digestion are possibly the most crucial of the body's activities, for it is on these cycles that all others depend. Without food of the proper nature, the body begins to ingest itself, and eventually, running out of substance, ceases to exist.

The cycles of digestion have evolved over thousands of years. The timing of these cycles is vital for optimal efficiency of our systems, and the Plan schedule respects this timing. Even though it takes some getting used to, just remember: It takes twenty-one days to change a habit! My clients feel so much better, are so much more connected in body and mind, and have so much more energy when they follow the Plan-designated times for eating.

Recently, a client's husband asked me if I could please make my system a little more flexible timewise to extend the evening dinner hours to around nine o'clock. I laughed when he asked me this! If you understand the cycles of digestion and how locked into human physiology they are, you'll laugh too, because what seems like a practical suggestion for convenience is actually tantamount to attempting to change the tides.

Timing Is Everything

Although the digestive system is able to perform all its functions all the time, the following time periods represent the best scenario for the cycles' optimum efficiency. When we eat at times that coordinate with digestive cycles, we support the body; in turn, the cycles become more effective in their action. To pick up on the Maserati metaphor, following this schedule is like having a very efficient motor in your car so that it drives with more energy, more speed, and the cleaner burning of fuel.

Elimination Cycle: 4 a.m. to 11 a.m.

Thorough elimination is a key element of the body's housecleaning before it begins the next eating cycle. Breakfast plays an important role, not only in creating energy for the day but also in easing the body into the elimination cycle. Breakfast should be energy-creating, not energy-taking; accordingly, heavy foods in the morning are not recommended except for individuals with already high metabolic burning rates.

It is important to understand that eating heavy foods between 4 a.m. and 8 a.m. compromises both the effectiveness of your elimination cycle and the next phase of digestion. Ineffective elimination also causes a condition called autointoxication, or "self-poisoning."

Eating late at night causes a similar distortion in the digestive process. The digestive process slows down in the evening and during sleep, therefore much of the food we eat late at night is incompletely digested. It is stored as fat or not assimilated properly, so it gets stuck somewhere in the process to allow the more important process of assimilation to continue. In general, the effectiveness of both assimilation and elimination is compromised. Notice that when you eat late, you do not have the same quality of energy in the morning.

Appropriation Cycle: 11 a.m. to 7 p.m.

The appropriation cycle takes place when food can be processed most efficiently for use in the body. Our energy is highest at midday, and that's when the digestive furnace can burn best.

NOTES

In many parts of the world, people have their main meal of the day at midday, taking time out to eat and relax before going back to work. Since the height of the digestive cycle occurs at that time, it's a logical time to have your heaviest meal and relax a little before returning to work. Many French, Italian, and Spanish people, for example, cling to their three-hour lunches, local food, and cultural cuisine in spite of changing economic times and the demands of North American business. The "Slow Food" movement started in resistance to these demands for the fast food and fast living of Western culture. Wikepedia defines Slow Food as "an international movement founded by Carlo Petrini in 1986. Promoted as an alternative to fast food, it strives to preserve traditional and regional cuisine and encourages farming of plants, seeds, and livestock characteristic of the local ecosystem."

Many North American travelers who return from Europe say that people really know how to live there. What they see as living fully is taking time out during the day to eat and rest as well as work. It's interesting how this daily ritual of a long, relaxing lunch sets a cultural standard. It shows a respect for the body and for oneself by reserving a regular part of every day to commune, relax, and enjoy food and life.

In the Western world and other countries eager to become westernized, the American model has been adopted. Taking time at midday involves too many moneymaking daylight hours, so we arc driven to eating on the run, grabbing a fifteen-minute or half-hour lunch, or gobbling fast food at our desk or in the car. Some companies order in "business lunches" of pizza or sandwiches, chips, and sodas to supposedly make better use of time, not waste it.

My friend's mother owns a restaurant in Geneva, Switzerland. It is a lovely place, with dark wood, good wines, excellent cuisine, and great service. I always marvel at the businessmen and bankers who show up for a pleasant lunch with their associates and order several courses of exquisite food,

> **The Plan is *not* a diet. It's a way of combining foods (the Tao of Eating, if you will)—the most sensible, unique, and fun weight-reduction program in this world. Each meal is a blessing of satisfaction and fulfillment in more ways than just eating. If you follow the Plan, results will be produced—fact, not fiction!**
> — *Sheila D., Designer*

leisurely consume a bottle of wine, and spend a few hours eating, drinking, and discussing business over their meal, which is fully appreciated and easily digested.

When we don't take time to eat well during the day, it's hard for us to get proper nutrition, and in the end, our body loses out. We miss the perfect digestive opportunity of the midday break, our energy flags in the afternoon, and by three o'clock we need a nap, a snack, or a caffeine fix.

Assimilation Cycle: 7 p.m. to 4 a.m.

The body is a miraculous creation. How it processes the raw materials we eat into extremely efficient fuel and building material can be truly inspiring—if we would just give it a chance.

The assimilation cycle of digestion is when nutrition happens, and it is the most crucial cycle for our body's health and well-being. It is the process of slowing down while our body works to process food into a form that can be used as fuel. Eating after 7 p.m. reduces our body's ability to extract nutritional value from what we give it to work with.

The body breaks down the raw materials of food with acids, enzymes, internal massage, fluid, and oxygenation. This creates the amino acids and sugars that the body, through osmosis and diffusion, can then assimilate into the bloodstream from the stomach and intestinal walls. The leftover products are siphoned through to the lower bowel for elimination.

If the body is in good shape and has successfully digested healthful food efficiently, all is well. It can then manage the constant rebuilding of cells and maintenance of energy beautifully. However, if assimilation is not optimal because of unsound food quality and choices,

NOTES

the organs can suffer with disturbances too numerous to list. If this is an ongoing state of affairs, the body's inability to process food effectively is impaired and nutrition is depleted, which creates a ripple effect that ends in breakdown. This breakdown leads directly to dysfunction and disease.

But I Work until Five O'clock

In our Western society, there are many reasons for eating late. Many commute long distances, stay late at work, take children to activities, or go to the gym—all considered more important than traditional dinnertime. Young children are hungry by early evening, so we try to feed them by 5 or 6. And it's interesting that in seniors' homes, dinner is still served regularly at 5:30. Why—when we make an effort to feed our children when they are hungry, and the elderly at times that work best for the body—do we feel those times don't apply to us?

Without proper nutrition and a stable eating environment, the quick mind and well-tuned body needed to accomplish and learn will deteriorate. There are a thousand justifiable reasons for why we don't eat at times that would support our body's cycles; however, those reasons are from the outside, not the inside, of our body and mind.

Your inner needs are what require your attention. Simply put, practical issues have to be reorganized. Instead of always shifting mealtimes to make things convenient for everything else, shift everything else around to accommodate the times your body needs to eat so you can start to enjoy optimal health. If

you try this, you'll be amazed to find that you may begin to run your life rather than your life always running you.

Ten O'clock: Our Natural Bedtime

Early to bed and early to rise makes a man healthy, wealthy, and wise.

— Benjamin Franklin (1706–1790)

Every hour we spend sleeping before midnight gives our body twice the value of every hour after midnight. Building a reasonable bedtime into your life, combined with eating meals at times that work for your body, boosts the functioning of your endocrine glands. Perhaps, then, your pineal gland will start to deliver the appropriate dose of melatonin you need for a sound night's sleep.

If you are a night owl, start gradually and work your bedtime back fifteen minutes each night. You'll notice a major difference in both the quantity and quality of your energy over a few months. At the beginning you might need an herbal tincture such as valerian, poppy, skullcap, or passionflower, and in addition a calcium and magnesium supplement for their calming and de-stressing effects (check with your doctor before using herbal or dietary supplements to make sure you have no medical condition or are taking any prescription medications that would conflict with them). Be patient and before too long your sleeping pills will become a thing of the past.

Note: Teenagers work on a different schedule, as many of you parents may have noticed. They are still in the maturing cycles, and as the acclaimed science writer Jennifer Ackerman says in her book *Sex Sleep Eat Drink Dream*, teenagers' going to bed later and sleeping into the day may not be as indulgent as you may have thought.

Cycling with the Moon

In one of the systems I was trained in, women's menstrual cycles are considered to be in tune with nature as well. If a woman is healthy and in her reproductive prime, her menstrual cycle usually begins on a full moon. Her ovulation is also in cycle with the moon and the tides and falls on the new moon. Some women ovulate on the full moon and begin their period on the new moon; either pattern is healthy. Many women, due to their choice of birth control method, do not have periods at all. Although convenient for our fast-paced lifestyle, putting off cycling is not something

I ever advise, since I have seen many of the side effects of long-term use of such pharmaceuticals. It can take a woman's body years to recover from such harsh, unnatural changes. Some women who stop taking these drugs in order to become pregnant often have difficulty ovulating again.

The natural timing of the menstrual cycle is something we do not want to fool with. Some cycles are longer than others, some shorter, some periods are heavier, some less so. Respecting and supporting the natural and regular female cycle is the focus that I would like to stress. Sometimes herbs are needed, sometimes glandulars, and sometimes just a structured, stress-reduced lifestyle. Remember Gaia, good old Mother Earth, is female, and female beings are a reflection of her cycles and her state of well-being.

NOTES

Change

CHAPTER FOUR

How We Resist Change

To many people, the thought of change seems threatening at first. Yet, this apprehension, which is only natural, is based on the illusion that change means loss of control. This couldn't be further from the truth. Change is what life is all about and when we surrender to that fact, we can, for the most part, be the pilots of our own lives and steer our own vessels. When we accept change instead of fighting it, we master the skill of making changes of our own choosing.

> — Dr. Christiane Northrup,
> *Women's Bodies, Women's Wisdom*

There are three basic ways that we tend to handle change: dissipating the energy, blocking the energy, and distracting from the energy. Each incorporates resistance. In his book *Thresholds of the Mind*, Bill Harris describes these three methods that we use to avoid being pushed over our threshold for change. Each of us has our particular coping mechanism, or a combination of these mechanisms, to avoid confronting and dealing with the discomfort of change.

1. Dissipating the Energy: Some people, when stressed or overwhelmed, frantically try to push change away through anger, crying, physical activity, sex, talking, or anything else that seems to stop the change and momentarily relieve the pressure.

2. Blocking the Energy: Others will do anything they can to avoid the change by isolating themselves, shutting down,

becoming depressed, or getting sick.

3. Distraction: The two strategies above are usually complemented by distraction with alcohol, drugs, sex, visual distractions such as TV and the Internet, exercise, or reading voraciously.

Not to get too scientific here, but if you really want to understand change and the strategies to prevent yourself from being a push-button machine to your reactors, you will need to have an understanding of entropy. Simply put, in an open system—of which human beings are a part—over time, all things tend to break down and become less ordered unless energy is added in some way. In other words, in all processes, including personal growth and lifestyle changes, energy gets lost and disorder and chaos result unless effort, focus, and energy are consistently added in.

We either eventually surrender to change or we suffer because of the long-term resistance to it. The less we resist, the less time we suffer. These conditions apply to all open systems in the universe. Resistance to change equals suffering.

Does that mean that if we just take things as they are we won't suffer? *Yes!* We resist only when the mind does not feel safe, and we don't feel safe when our patterns of safety, developed during childhood, and which often no longer make sense, are threatened. How can we feel safe? As silly as it may sound, have a little chat with yourself and make a promise that you will only do things that will ensure your safety.

The principles of the Plan will help you feel safe. Eating in accordance with the forces and timing of nature works. Doing the things that work for your body and mind, such as breathing and chewing and moving in a structured way, works. The body and mind love structure; a feeling of safety is often the result.

The First Step to Feeling Safe and Working with Resistance

It's truly a sight to see when the inhabitants of any planetary civilization cross the tipping point and begin to individually accept complete and eternal responsibility for their own happiness. Yet, this hardly compares to the mountain-quaking, body-shaking, polarity-flipping, hero-making occurrences that transpire when such inhabitants graduate to accepting complete and eternal responsibility for their every twinge of unhappiness. Brings tears to my eyes.

— Mike Dooley, *Notes from the Universe*

Suffering is generated through attraction and aversion, and there is usually emotion connected to them. We are attracted or drawn strongly to happiness or to averting and avoiding pain. If we can remain in the present moment and just notice the attraction or aversion and not be drawn into it, suffering will not occur.

Fear and hope are the continuum that creates suffering. They involve fear of loss and hope for gain, fear of blame and hope for praise, fear of infamy and hope for fame, fear of pain and hope for pleasure.

Exercise in Observation

Notice, just notice, what happens to you when you are faced with a change and do not do anything about it. Watch your resistance, your attitudes, your thoughts, and your body responses and allow them to be just as they are.

Learning to observe can take time, but you

will master it, and then nothing will hook you. You will become calm in all situations, since your well-being will not be in danger; you will be like an actor in a movie of your choice, responding as you choose.

Many people think this sounds plastic and unreal, but the truth is, being affected by your emotions and circumstances is really what is plastic and unreal. You are then a robot at the beck and call of every media mogul, every eye-catching girl or guy, every mouth-watering piece of cake, every tear-jerking soap opera.

We are hooked on stimulation and emotion, negative or positive. Every time someone or something wants to control you, they just push button L and you laugh, button C and you cry, button A and you get angry, button D and you get depressed. Truly, is this a live, fully expressive human being who is able to choose how and why he or she participates in life? Doesn't sound that way to me.

Does just being an observer make you feel distant or bored? Just observing can make you feel calm and peaceful, because you are choosing how you experience a situation; you are engaged, not bored. We are so afraid of being bored. We are constantly being stimulated in our society, so boredom can feel like dying. If there is no resistance, boredom is calming.

Observing and choosing which stimuli to participate in is not boring; it is the ultimate power to choose. The juice here is that when you participate, you are fully in the experience and a full partner to your reality. Now *that* is juicy!

So, when you are present and not caught in the fear, hope, and resistance paradigm, sex is better, food is exquisite, exercise is bliss, sunsets are stunning, love is rapture, all by choice. No robot here!

Tools to deal with resistance are necessary, and building them into your everyday way of

NOTES

being is a necessary part of moving forward. The ability to notice when you are resisting is the first step; you could call it being in a state of observation rather than reaction.

Feeling Safe and Dealing with Resistance

The ability to observe does not happen overnight. In Chapter Six, "Coaxing Metabolism," I provide you with some tools that will support you in the process. However, in the meantime, here are some actions to help you get through the muck when you encounter resistance.

Often resistance feels as though your feet are stuck in molasses, or your head is fuzzy and you can't think straight. Resistance shows up in many ways; you have your own particular style. When you notice that you want to run, or are about to use any of the strategies to avoid change—dissipating or blocking energy or finding a distraction—try to catch yourself and do one or all of the following three actions:

1. **Breathe**: The first action is to breathe. In Chapter Two, "Habits," I told you about the importance of breath and moving blocked wind energy. This method definitely applies to resistance. Whenever you find yourself resisting, breathe. Paying attention and catching yourself in your thought pattern, and then breathing through it can be done in all situations; no matter what you are doing, where you are, or whatever the circumstances, breathe.

2. **Move**: The second action is exercise, and the best solution to resistance may be walking. In addition, in Chapter Eight, "Movement," I present a set of metabolic exercises, yogic in nature, to help you cope in

body and mind with the changes you are making to your lifestyle, including the way you react to emotional stimulation. Move your feet through that molasses!

3. **Communicate**: The third action is to communicate. Let it go, let someone support you. That does not mean dumping your emotional load on someone else; it is simply letting someone else hear you. You can communicate with a coach (me, or a coach I have trained), either in person, by phone, or by email, or with a friend or partner. You can communicate with a buddy who is doing this new lifestyle plan with you and can support you—rather than agree with you. It may just be a friend with good ears who can keep quiet and nod a lot. Being heard is one of the most effective ways to make resistance dissipate and stop you from diving into your normal coping mechanisms. It opens the door to transformation and change. There is no fixing here, just being heard is sufficient. Let's call it re-creation. When you hear yourself in someone else's listening, you will hear yourself and the situation differently. And what is really great (if that person is a good listener), is that all your concerns about the situation you are talking about will disappear.

Noticing and Observing, and That's All

In all cases involving resistance, it is necessary that you have enough distance from your story to at least see what you are doing. Most of the time when we are going through change, we are a push-button reaction machine and fall into one or more of our coping strategies without thinking at all. We just fall in.

To catch ourselves, we need to be present and aware of what is going on right now! This is called mindfulness or mindful awareness. Then all you do is notice and observe—and not fix! (I discuss mindfulness in Chapter Nine, "Communication.")

Loving Kindness

In order to get to the point of noticing, you have to care enough and have enough compassion for yourself to do just that. You need loving kindness toward yourself to notice, instead of trying to fix a situation or pulling out the big stick from the closet (where you keep it handy) to beat yourself about the head and shoulders for making yet another mistake, for not living up to your, your mother's, your father's, your boss's, your kids', or whoever else's standards. Don't even go to the closet. Just notice. (See Chapter Nine, "Communication" for a daily practice in loving kindness.)

Adjusting to Change

It is difficult to give up old habits and drop sugar and stimulant addictions to help you regain well-being. The body has to make many adjustments to change; for example, just in temperature alone the body has to adjust to swings in both internal (body temperature) and external (weather) changes. Therefore,

NOTES

we need to have respect and compassion for our body as it copes with change, not just physical changes such as temperature but also major lifestyle changes like the one you are about to embark on.

Change is difficult and causes upset. If you think that change is easy, just try a little experiment. Each evening turn off your phone, computer, and TV. Run a warm bath with bath salts and essential oils. Light scented candles, put on quiet music, and soak for an hour. Do this little ritual for a week. On the eighth day, don't do it. You will feel robbed and cheated mentally, emotionally, and physically. You will react to the change, and so will your body—and that was only a week, not a lifetime. Learning to listen to what your body is saying as it goes through change is a part of your new lifestyle plan.

> **What I loved most about this plan, then, and what keeps me on it three years and a fourth child later, is how it has taught me to listen very closely to what my body tells me it needs. Sometimes it whispers, and sometimes it shouts (I can be very stubborn), but I've learned that there are certain 'rules' that govern my body's functioning at an optimum level. I know with amazing accuracy exactly which foods I can or should not indulge in, and I can predict the precise consequences of ignoring those rules.**
> — *Susan W., Arbonne Distributor, Wife and Mother*

The Voice of the Body

Many individuals who have jumped into the Plan are consistently startled, and pleasantly surprised, by some of their reactions to change:

- Sugar cravings, even for sweetaholics and chocaholics, disappear in the first four days (the rest is in your head).
- Reflux, heartburn, and digestive discomfort are relieved almost immediately.
- Energy starts to build quickly.
- Happiness shows up unexpectedly.
- When they begin to chew and breathe, taste buds pop; food tastes wonderful.
- Time stretches to allow time to eat meals slowly.

Body Talk

When you begin to listen, your body starts to talk to you. It tells you what foods it likes and what volumes of food work. It tells you whether you got enough sleep and if you are following the program properly. Over time, you will learn not to listen to your demanding ego trying to overpower the conversation, but to the soft, clear voice of your body demonstrating its needs. It does happen.

When you listen to your body, you will have a new respect for it, as you realize the many trials you had put it through with your unconscious demands over the years. For those of you who have listened too hard and become compulsive, you can begin to ease up and give yourself a little freedom; loosen up a bit. No matter where you and your body have come from, compassion will show up loud and clear as you train yourself to listen and have compassion for your body.

Your appetite may take awhile to catch up with the process, but when it does, it is an indicator that the digestive system and metabolism are beginning to wake up to their real functions. Blood sugar may take awhile, too. You may find you still need a cup of black tea in the afternoon to get through without your energy flagging too much. But it will come.

NOTES

Chemistry

The doctor of the future will give no medicine, but will interest his patients in the care of the human frame, in diet, and in the cause and prevention of disease.

— Thomas Edison, American Inventor
(1847–1931)

I was never very good at math. When I started high-school chemistry, a large part of which was math, I was totally at a loss because of the math skills required to understand chemistry.

To his credit, my chemistry teacher could teach anyone—he would take you right into the natural world and show you how it worked. Mr. Kendall owned an orchard and did a lot of grafting. He would take us there to look at the grafts, and then back in the classroom lab he would teach us the chemistry behind what made two plant parts successfully join as one. His grafts produced some unusual species of flowers and fruit. Seeing chemistry with a biochemistry focus diminished my phobia. Understanding how chemistry made things work was exciting, and it proved to be exciting again and again over time.

Since that time, I have discovered that everything in the human body is chemistry. The dance of the molecules at the cellular level; the profound effects of DNA; and the fine-tuned precision of hormones, enzymes, acids, diffusion, and osmosis are all fascinating. When I see these phenomena working in unique ways in each individual's body, I find the subject even more interesting, and the challenge of helping the individual find balance in body and mind is what keeps me doing what I do.

Food, minerals, water, assimilation, together with cell construction and the composition of the chemical juice it requires, have a huge role to play in the internal dance of the elements. The mind also plays a large part in the control of the acid-alkaline (pH) balance of our blood and other fluids, as well as the control of our emotional reactions, hormone balance, expenditure of physical energy, oxygenation, and hydration.

The Plan is designed to set up and maintain the fine-tuned symphony of internal metabolic chemistry in each individual. It is the way to get that wonderfully well-designed Maserati back into tip-top performance.

Enzymes

Each type of food we eat (protein, starch, fat, and fiber) has a matching enzyme to help digest and assimilate it effectively. Without these enzymes we would not survive: The food we eat would not be digested properly, and therefore we would not have the raw materials for our body to repair itself and function normally. The body produces these enzymes, but sometimes supplementary enzymes can help with digestive problems.

The Role of Enzymes as We Age

In later life, you may have noticed, people often grow to look like skin and bone. They may have fat on their body, yet it looks different and less well distributed than when they were younger. As we grow older, hormones change

and reduce in intensity. So do enzymes. By the time most of us reach our seventies, our enzyme and stomach acid intensity is reduced by up to seventy-five percent. Our enzyme production begins reducing at the ripe age of twenty-seven. What does this mean to our digestion?

It means we need to either use supplements for digestive support—or become younger. Some things need to be augmented as we age. For some of us, these things are hormones, and for most of us, they are enzymes, acids, and probiotics, the latter to maintain the fine balance of internal flora in our intestines. Supplementing at this basic level of the digestive chain guarantees better digestive function, acid-alkaline balance, and energy production in the short and the long term. It guarantees more of our food ends up as energy used as it was meant to be, not built up as fat in our arteries or as misplaced minerals in our joints. Supplementation can come from food that is high in enzymes, such as cultured food.

Enzyme support can come from food combining and cultured food and by avoiding foods that makes digestion difficult. I discuss food combining and cultured and fermented foods later in this chapter.

Digestive Acids

Hydrochloric acid (HCl) is one of those substances in the body that is often badly maligned but that does not deserve its reputation. Heartburn and reflux are so present in daily life that they have become commonplace. Antacids sell over the counter and by prescription, and many people take these medicines to reduce acidity, when the problem is often actually the reverse—a lack of acid needed for proper digestion.

The miraculous digestive juices are first activated in the mouth by adequate chewing. When food is not well chewed, the body must deliver large spurts of acid to dissolve the insufficiently masticated food. The body's acid becomes depleted because of this increased demand. Depleted HCl is very common.

When individuals begin eating in the Plan fashion, they sometimes require HCl and pancreatic enzymes to straighten out these deficiencies. Once the acid and enzymes are re-regulated, these individuals can back off on the supplementation and use HCl and enzymes only with very heavy protein meals or not at all.

Eighty percent of people who get onto the Plan are off their antacids and digestive aids within a week. The other twenty percent have more serious digestive problems, so they must be supported with supplementation for a while, but not forever. Eventually, our body recovers its ability to digest food when we remove our stressors; when we eat, chew, and breathe properly; and when we give our system a chance to recover with cultured food and food combining.

If we would just breathe, sit down, chew, and combine our food properly, then there would be little or no need for the digestive drugs. I will not go into detail about the effects of pharmaceutical drugs on digestion, assimilation, and energy, but there are profound systemic limitations resulting from the ingestion of certain pharmaceuticals. The ones that are most commonly prescribed are blood pressure medications; cholesterol

NOTES

medications, such as statins; arthritis, thyroid, and diabetic supports (for those not on insulin); antibiotics; steroids; pain medications; and antacid prescriptions. These drugs often contribute to older people's being unable to digest, assimilate, and eliminate well, since they change digestive chemistry.

Drugs are useful in the case of an emergency, or if a physical condition gets out of control, but most drugs can be used for the immediate emergency and then be replaced with proper nutrition, lifestyle change, and supplements. This does not apply in all cases, but in a high percentage of cases.

Internal Flora

Disease states often begin with an imbalance of flora in the intestinal tract. This can be caused by emotional or physical distress (including adrenal fatigue); hormone imbalance or pharmaceutical drugs, especially antibiotics; birth control pills; and steroids. A few common conditions that require a probiotic supplement include vomiting, diarrhea, and stomach flu, or overuse of alcohol, simple starches, or sugar. Adding ongoing dietary support (e.g., organic plain yogurt, kefir, cultured fruit and vegetables, and kombucha tea) to daily food intake helps to regenerate and maintain balanced internal flora in a world of daily exposure to emotional and environmental stressors.

Food Combining: Don't Eat Foods That Fight

Dr. William Hay introduced food combining in 1911. He had several clinics and consulted with health spas in Europe and the United Kingdom that were treating health disorders with nutrition, baths, rest, and alkalizing minerals. The premise held by Dr. Hay was that the underlying cause of illness and disease was an imbalance of chemistry in the body. This condition was caused by excess acidity, a by-product of the digestive process and lifestyle imbalances. His theory was that alkalinity in the body keeps it balanced and well and acidity creates a propensity for a higher inflammatory response, which damages organs and tissues and reduces the general functioning of the body.

The message that people took away from Dr. Hay's healing spas was, "Don't eat foods that fight." Since that time, many books have made this theory both effective and popular. Harvey and Marilyn Diamond's *Fit for Life* and Joel Fuhrman's *Eat to Live* are examples of books that support food combining. Many practitioners have supported this theory with a great deal of success. Teachers with whom I studied used it as a cornerstone of their practice and teaching: Rev. Hanna Kroeger of Boulder, Colorado, and her assistant Bobbi Brooks from New Albany, Indiana, as well as Dr. Tipps, a naturopath from Austin, Texas.

In the food chain, each food classification has a digestive enzyme that resonates with it and helps the body digest that food with particular efficiency. Enzymes break down the food to be digested so that the body can convert it for energy, growth, and repair. Some foods and their enzyme partners work well with other foods and their enzymes, and others do not, thus we have foods that fight and foods that work in harmony.

Foods that harmonize are proteins and complex carbohydrates; meat, poultry, and fish digest well with complex carbohydrates such as kale, broccoli, spinach, and other non-starchy vegetables. Whole grains require more digestive time than simple starches such as refined grains. Dairy products digest well with proteins and nonstarchy vegetables such as tomatoes and pickled cucumbers. Fats and oils digest well with proteins, complex carbohydrates, and dairy products. Starchy vegetables such as potatoes, and whole grains such as brown rice, whole-grain bread, and whole-grain pasta digest well with all vegetables. Fruits digest best on their own, at least two hours away from all other foods.

Following are some examples of meals made up of good food combinations:

- Grilled fish, broccoli, and a green salad with an oil-based dressing (no starches or fruit)
- Whole-grain, wheat-free/gluten-free pasta with tomato sauce; grilled zucchini; and a green salad (no oil or butter, cheese or meat)
- Fresh fruit plate (at least two hours away from other foods)

Cultured and fermented drinks such as kefir and kombucha tea, in addition to cultured or fermented vegetables and fruit such as sauerkraut, pickled daikon radish, and umeboshi plums can be eaten with proteins, fats, and starches. Because of their high enzyme concentration, they are able to break down difficult food combinations and help combat problems of yeast overgrowth such as candida. Taken after a badly combined meal, the cultures help the body deal with the chal-

NOTES

lenge by making digestion more effective and eliminating bloating, gas, and heartburn.

Three meals a day, about four hours apart, follows the natural processing rhythm of the body. This pattern is recommended in many books about food combining because it optimizes the body's processing ability. Food combining and eating three meals a days alone can result in the elimination of digestive problems, including heartburn, reflux, gas, and bloating. There is often a dramatic increase in energy, and the body often becomes a leaner, more efficient burning machine.

Note: The exception to these rules of food combining in this approach is the breakfast. (I explain the rationale behind that in the section "Breakfast and the Boil" in Chapter Six.)

Getting back to the Maserati metaphor: If you want to have a clean, sleek machine that runs at optimum all the time, then you'll want to give it fuel in combinations that are easy for the engine to burn. The same applies to getting your metabolic system functioning efficiently. If you give your body food it can digest efficiently and with more ease than usual, you will produce cleaner energy and have more

> **At my first appointment with Rae, I quickly realized I knew less than I thought about which foods were good for me and which foods were not. Many of the foods I thought were good for me were actually counter-productive to my goals.**
> — *Bruce M.*

energy available whenever you need it.

Mono Meals

Another theory that follows food combining in principle is that of mono meals. Eating just one food at a time makes digestion almost effortless. It eases up the digestive process so the body can get nourishment, yet concentrates on whatever healing and antibody production is most needed at the time. If the body has undergone a particularly stressful period due to illness, trauma, surgery, or exhaustion, eating mono meals is a way to offer little holidays for the system. It is a style of fasting.

Cultured and Fermented Foods

Most ethnic groups throughout history have included fermented foods and drinks in their diet that are usually consumed with every meal. The lactobacilli in fermented drinks and foods help to promote the growth of beneficial bacteria in the intestines, as well as offering enzymes that support digestion. These foods have been used for centuries to provide relief from gas and bloating, overwork, overeating, and overuse of alcohol.

Here are some examples of fermented

foods from around the world:

- Japan: Pickled umeboshi plums and pickled vegetables
- Switzerland: Swiss herbal stomach bitters and yogurt
- Germany and the Netherlands: Sauerkraut and pickled vegetables
- Russia: Kombucha tea, sour cream, borscht, and kvass (fermented grain or beet juice)
- India: Pickled vegetables, lassi (salty or sweet yogurt drink)
- France: *Fromage blanc* (fresh, unripened cheese)
- Middle Eastern countries: Ayran (salty yogurt drink)
- Aboriginals in the South American Andes have fermented berry drinks, which, although also mildly psychogenic or alcoholic, support beneficial intestinal flora.

Adding some of these alternative digestives are a tasty addition to the diet, and a tremendous support for any time you find your system feels sluggish. Your body will respond immediately to their healing effects by moving the bowels and improving digestion.

Fermented products are a vibrant source of protein that can spice up your food. Although I am not in favor of soy as a staple, fermented soy products such as tempeh and wheat-free/gluten-free tamari offer many health benefits. Although *natto* (fermented soybeans) does not appeal to me personally, it does sell well, so there must be quite a few people who like it.

Note: People who have been dependent on unfermented soy products (such as tofu or soy protein) seem to recover their energy

NOTES

quickly when they remove them from their diet. Unfermented soy products are known to cause many health problems, including disrupting thyroid function, as described in Kaayla Daniel's book *The Whole Soy Story*.

Kombucha Tea

Although many people are under the impression that kombucha is a mushroom, it is actually a bacterium. The name *kombucha* may sound like a mushroom, its appearance may be the color of a mushroom, and the fermenting bacterium may have a mushroom look to it when it is growing, but kombucha is definitely a bacterium. As such, it's a good digestive aid and an excellent source of probiotics. I recommend it for people with a compromised immune system or with severe digestive problems.

The kombucha culture is originally from a Russian recipe and they can multiply quickly. Known as *scobies*, the cultures are shared among neighbors. You can add ginger and fruit to your kombucha tea for flavor, and you can add sugar, honey, and green or black tea to the scoby. Because the sugar burns up in the process of fermentation, it is not particularly sweet. Effervescent and a little sharp, the tea can have quite a kick to it. Bottled kombucha tea is available in some health food stores, but often it is sweetened with cane sugar, so read the labels before purchasing. Added sugars may appeal to the taste buds, but kombucha tea is meant to aid digestion and not to be just a tasty drink. Here is a standard recipe for kombucha tea:

Kombucha Tea

4 cups (1 L) filtered water
¼ cup (60 mL) sugar
1 tablespoon (15 mL) loose black or green tea, or 2 teabags
½ cup (125 mL) kombucha culture (scoby)

Combine the water and sugar in a saucepan and bring it to a boil over medium-high heat. Turn off the heat and add the tea. Cover and let sit for 15 minutes.

Strain the tea into a glass bowl and set aside to cool to room temperature, and then place the culture in the liquid. (Reserve the liquid in which your culture came.) Cover the bowl with a cloth and store it in a warm place for a few days to a week. Taste the liquid; it is ready when it is less sweet and reaches your desired acidity.

The skin that forms on the top is your new culture. Transfer it to the reserved liquid from the first culture. Store your kombucha in the refrigerator.

Sprouting

Sprouting is a great way to increase your protein intake (especially if you're vegetarian); reduce your body's acidity; and get the nourishment of young, raw, fresh green vegetables. It's simple and easy to do at home. Soak the seeds of any vegetable on a sprouting tray (please see the Resources section) until they "wake up" and sprout. Eating sprouts will definitely give your body a great wakeup too! These micro-vegetables have high concentrations of protein and can nourish vegetarians and anyone who has difficulty digesting heavier animal proteins.

Each sprout has its own unique flavor. Some are mild, others peppery, some sharp, some spicy. Experiment with radish, mung beans, broccoli, peas, and many more—the variety is almost unlimited. Sprouts can also bring your salads to life and add flavor to your cooked dishes. Just have fun with them. Raw nuts and seeds can be sprouted as well.

Diseases such as cancer and autoimmune dysfunction benefit greatly from the addition of these easily digested sources of protein.

NOTES

The Science of Alternating Foods

Alternating types of meals to stimulate digestion is another way to re-regulate the body. When the body is forced to come up with a new strategy for the digestion of each meal, it has to shift and alter its metabolic response. Basically, the body must change gears, which stimulates function. Alternating between a meal of mostly animal protein and a meal of mostly starch, or an all-fruit meal, challenges the body to digest, making it dig for the resources to do so. This is good. It may take a little time to become accustomed to this style of eating, but it quickly becomes an energizing new habit.

Protein Meals

Over fifty percent of lunches or dinners on the Plan are high in protein, since it is this factor that stimulates the thyroid, increases metabolic response, and helps to burn fat. A typical Plan meal would consist of baked chicken breast with mushroom sauce, steamed broccoli with butter, cooked carrots, a large green salad with oil and lemon dressing, cheese slices, and a glass of white wine.

During the first phase of the Plan, protein intake is high, but once metabolic function is normalized and consistent, the consumption of protein can be reduced to approximately twenty-five percent of the protein meal.

Starch Meals

Starch meals should be included in the repertoire three to four times a week, alternating them with meat, poultry, or fish and vegeta-

ble meals (never have a starch meal for both lunch and dinner in the same day).

Here are some examples of starch meals. Notice that they do not include fat, oils, dairy, or animal protein.

- Boiled potatoes, steamed broccoli, and a green salad with Dijon mustard and apple cider vinegar dressing (the dressing can also be put on the potatoes).
- Quinoa pasta with strained tomatoes, steamed zucchini, *herbes de Provence*, and a sliced tomato salad with wasabi and rice vinegar dressing.
- Short-grain brown rice with steamed broccoli, yellow zucchini, and chopped Swiss chard with umeboshi plum vinegar.

You will find many other easy recipes for starch meals in the pasta section of my cookbook *The Alive Recipe Collection: Sculpting Your Body with Food.*

Fruit Meals Too

Having meals of only fruit to alter digestive rates and enzyme response is also an option. Please make sure it is a day with a light agenda and low activity (I usually choose Sunday), since fruit meals do not last long in the system and you will become tired and hungry more quickly than if you have protein, or even starches, in your stomach. Eating bananas and berries while on a car trip is a good time for this kind of meal. Cooked fruit, such as fruit compote, is another option. (I have a delicious cooked-fruit recipe in "The Boil" section of *The Alive Recipe Collection.*)

My favorite Sunday brunch meal is always a banana smoothie. Here's a recipe you can try:

Banana Smoothie

Yield: 1 serving

4 to 6 ripe bananas, coarsely chopped

1 handful each of strawberries, blueberries, blackberries, and raspberries

½ teaspoon (2.5 mL) ground cinnamon

½ teaspoon (2.5 mL) ground cloves

½ teaspoon (2.5 mL) ground nutmeg

1 cup (250 mL) cold water

1 cup (250 mL) crushed ice

Put the bananas, berries, cinnamon, cloves, and nutmeg in a blender. Add the water and process until smooth. Stir in the crushed ice and serve. Drink slowly and enjoy!

NOTES

Coaxing Metabolism

CHAPTER SIX

Foods to Eliminate

Our goal with this plan is to make the metabolic system a smooth-running, energy-efficient machine. It can be difficult to get the metabolism to gear up, so it makes sense to try to make it as easy and productive as we can by streamlining digestive function at the beginning of the program. To this end, in this chapter I list certain foods that I recommend eliminating during the first part of the Plan: Cleansing and Transition. You may not immediately see the justification for eliminating some of the foods on this list, but I assure you that the reasons are sound. I have explained briefly the reasons for many of the eliminations, some of which may come as quite a revelation.

As you begin to listen to the metabolic responses of your body, you may be surprised by your body's reaction when you eliminate them, and then again when you reintroduce them.

Having accomplished your goals during the Cleansing and Transition phase, you will have learned to listen to your body's signals. When you move on to the second part of the plan, Balance and Support, adding back one food at a time from the original elimination list (especially at the midday meal) for a minimum three-day trial, your body will let you know what works and what does not. Your body will be your gauge, and your newly developed skill in listening to its messages will let you see which foods it likes and those it does not.

FOODS TO ELIMINATE

Food	Reason for Eliminating
Asparagus	High in sugar; the asparagines in asparagus stimulate the kidneys; eliminate for the first part of the Plan
Beans and lentils	Legumes are difficult to digest; can cause gas and bloating
Bread	Have wheat-free/gluten-free bread only at breakfast, otherwise avoid it entirely; this starch digests too quickly and does not provide enough roughage to be used in other meals (also see "Against the Grain" below)
Cabbage, Brussels sprouts, and turnips	Difficult to digest; can cause gas and bloating
Chocolate	Causes a breakdown in the muscles of the lower esophagus, increasing the likelihood of heartburn and indigestion
Coffee	Sterols and caffeine in coffee interfere with thyroid hormone production
Distilled alcohol	Compromises all body systems, including digestion; poisons the liver and causes reduced endocrine hormone function; notable exceptions, because they are fermented beverages and not distilled alcohol, are red and white wine, champagne, cider, and wheat-free beer, which are permitted only with meals, provided you eat part of your meal before drinking
Garlic and onions	Not permitted raw or cooked; they disturb digestion, are overstimulating and high in sugar, and garlic is known to disturb brain chemistry
Margarine and other artificial fats with transfats	Transfats are toxic and cause arterial blockage

FOODS TO ELIMINATE (cont'd)

Food	Reason for Eliminating
Milk	All milk, including cow's or milk made with soy, hemp, or nuts, can be difficult to digest
Processed and deli-style meat	Must be eliminated; the preservatives nitrites, nitrates, sulfites, and sulfates cause arterial blockage and slow metabolic function
Radishes and cucumber	Can alter hormone function and digestion; can be eaten if they are naturally pickled
Soda pop, sports drinks (regular or diet)	These drinks contain bromines, preservatives, and additives; they can cause lymphatic congestion and weight gain
Sugar and sugar substitutes	Tend to overstimulate insulin production; includes all sugar substitutes (natural or otherwise); a notable exception is honey, which is used with cultured butter for breakfast, but only in the morning
Sweet potatoes	Too high in sugar and have a tendency to go moldy; eliminate for the first part of the Plan
Tropical fruit	These fruits digest too quickly and are too high in sugar for early in the Plan, avoid until the pancreas is better able to regulate sugar levels
Unfermented soy products	Unfermented soy products, such as tofu and soy milk, have been found to disturb thyroid function
White products	Avoid all refined salt, refined sugar, and refined (white) flour, since the processing uses chemicals that are detrimental to the body; there are no sugars on the Plan (also see "Shopping for Sugar" later in this chapter)

PERMITTED FOODS

Food	Notes
Bananas and berries	Permitted as a meal on their own
Cooked fruit	Apples, pears, berries, cherries, plums, apricots as a meal on their own
Dijon mustard, capers, artichokes, kosher dill pickles, roasted red peppers, canned tomatoes	Permitted if free of sugar, wheat, garlic, onion, and preservatives
Fermented soy products	Such as wheat-free/gluten-free tamari, tempeh, and natto
Fresh vegetable juices	Permitted as an appetizer with any meal, including breakfast
Gluten-free or low-gluten pasta	Such as rice, Ezekiel, quinoa, and corn pastas
Gluten-, sugar-, and sweetener-free crackers	Permitted only as an appetizer
Grapefruit and lemon	Permitted with any other foods
Raw organic almonds	Permitted with protein meals only

NOTES

Some other foods need to be discussed in more detail. They are gluten, sugar, soy, salt, garlic, and onions.

Against the Grain

Many children and adults are allergic to both gluten and soy, and some to the milk protein casein as well. As a result, many alternatives to gluten grains, vegetable protein, and dairy milk have been introduced to the marketplace over the past decade.

Gluten is a protein found in some grains, wheat in particular, that becomes elastic when made into dough for bread. This is the reason it is so practical and useful as a binder for flour products. Reactions to gluten can include gas, bloating, diarrhea, and digestive discomfort, as well as more subtle reactions such as headaches, edema, weight gain, sinus congestion, and constipation. People with ce-liac disease have extreme reactions to gluten, and people with this condition must always avoid all grains that contain gluten; these include wheat, rye, spelt, kamut, barley, and often oats. A high percentage of people are sensitive to wheat, but not to all grains that contain gluten. Their symptoms may be of the more subtle and less-easy-to-notice variety.

Celiac disease is a digestive condition triggered by gluten, and gluten grains are used in most commercial breads, pasta, cookies, cakes, pizza crusts, and many other baked goods. When a person with celiac disease eats foods containing gluten, an immune reaction occurs in the gut, resulting in damage to the lining of the intestines. As a result, the person cannot absorb many nutrients from their food. The obvious symptoms of celiac disease include abdominal pain, diarrhea, bloating,

NOTES

and intense discomfort.

Eventually, decreased absorption of nutrients can cause vitamin deficiencies that deprive the brain, nervous system, bones, liver, and the organs responsible for digestion, leading to other illnesses. The decreased nutrient absorption that occurs in celiac disease is especially serious in children, who need proper nutrition to develop and grow. No treatment has yet been found to cure celiac disease. However, you can effectively manage the condition through changing your diet. In counseling people for many years, I have seen that a surprising percentage of our population is sensitive to wheat, and often they are intolerant to gluten.

Our medical establishment is just becoming aware of celiac disease and starting to connect the dots around many misdiagnosed conditions that are actually an allergy to gluten. Fortunately, there are now more and more choices of gluten-free foods in our grocery stores.

The Plan is not officially gluten-free, but it is wheat-free, and therefore gluten-reduced. The Plan can be followed by people with celiac disease simply by eliminating the other gluten grain products: rye, barley, spelt, and kamut (and sometimes oats). Grains that have no gluten, such as rice, amaranth, millet, and quinoa, can be included in the food plan. For most of us, it is a case of eliminating wheat, a primary culprit in problematic digestive symptoms.

In my late twenties, I developed colitis. Colitis is a condition that may include pain,

tenderness in the abdomen, fever, swelling of the colon tissue, bleeding, rectal bleeding, bloody diarrhea, and ulcerations of the colon. Advanced or more severe conditions include ulcerative colitis and Crohn's disease, both of which come with more severe symptoms.

In dealing with colitis, I found that changing my diet and eliminating dairy and wheat had an immediate positive effect. As a result, I kept my diet wheat- and dairy-free for many years. Often milk intolerance and sensitivity to wheat are both symptoms of an overstressed immune system. Avoidance of certain foods and change of lifestyle helped me to rebuild a healthy immune system. Since that time, and even before developing the Plan, I have found that eliminating wheat and cow's milk from my clients' diets has proven to relieve stress-induced symptoms and immune-compromised systems.

Asian Bean: Friend or Foe?

Soybeans are relatively new to Western culture, but as with all things that look like a hardy new cash crop from Asia, and an especially cheap solution, since it is so versatile, soy became a popular food that was quickly overused as a food and as an additive.

Considering the price of grain, allergies to wheat and gluten, and the rising new strains of grain viruses, soybeans at first looked like manna from heaven. Soybeans are hardy and able to resist many of our existing bacterial and insect foes. They are also quite adaptable to our climate and growing conditions. Farmers jumped at the chance to grow this extremely versatile product, using it to replace their wheat, rye, corn, and tobacco crops. As a result, market demand grew from nil to astronomical levels in very few years.

Soy Alternative

Soy was the solution to milk allergy for baby formula, it was used as a food additive as a binder, and because of the isoflavones in soy, which have an estrogenic effect, it found its way to being a "natural" version of hormone replacement therapy. Components of soy had positive effects on cancer. Additionally, soy takes on the flavor of whatever it is mixed with, and it can be eaten in numerous forms: TVP (texturized vegetable protein), powdered soy protein, tofu, soy sauce, soy milk, soy oil, and on and on. As a result, the marketplace was deluged with soy within a few years of its introduction to the West.

As is often discovered about supposed solutions that are overapplied, there are side effects, and in the case of soy, these side effects began to show up in the early nineties. Even though it is not broadly publicized, bit by bit people are becoming educated about the negative aspects of soy.

Soy products were never meant to be eaten in excess. In countries such as China and Japan, soy sauce is added as a flavoring and used as a condiment, or small chunks of tofu are added to miso soup, but they don't use large slabs of tofu as a meat replacement, or make tofu cheesecake, for example, as we do in the West. In addition, Asians generally eat a much smaller volume of food than people in the West, especially North Americans. Soybeans, fermented soy, tofu, and other soy products have always been eaten sparingly in the East, and they have been used for thousands of years, so Easterners' digestive systems have

NOTES

accommodated soy, and they do not experience the adverse reactions that we in the West do. When nutrition experts use the health of Eastern cultures as a rationale for adding soy to everything, they are ignoring the truth.

In my observations as a health practitioner, some people do well on unfermented soy, but a large majority does not. Most people experience gas, bloating, hormonal changes, sluggishness, and mental fogginess, as well as an abundance of other side effects, including weight gain. There is no doubt that the phytoestrogens found in soy products can be beneficial to those who have an estrogen deficiency, but again, this may apply to some, not to all.

The jury is out on soy with regard to its effect on the thyroid gland, but there is definitely concern, even in the medical research community, about the effect of soy on metabolism. I have many women coming to me complaining of thyroid symptoms, including hormone imbalance, low energy, no libido, sluggish digestion, slow bowel function, and lymphatic distress or excessive swelling of the extremities. Many of these women have good results and some even experience immediate elimination of these symptoms when they are taken off soy, wheat, and milk products. In addition, most have found that adding soy back into their diet has had a negative effect on their energy. The conclusion is clear: Soy does have negative effects for some people.

Reports also assert that soy affects male reproductive ability. It is believed that some young boys have developed breasts and shrinking testes due to the estrogenic effects of soy.

However, I think this is also due to the excess of xenoestrogens in the environment, not just to the overuse of soy in everyday processed foodstuffs.

My recommendation is that while you are introducing yourself to the Plan, your soy intake be limited to fermented soy; that is, miso, tempeh, natto, and wheat-free/gluten-free tamari (soy sauce). Every other form of soy may have some impact on your success with the Plan.

Garlic and Onions? "But I Am Italian!"

Garlic and onions are commonly used for cooking in our Western culture, and like sugar, these ingredients are in most prepared and packaged foods. Interestingly, in the East garlic and onions are used quite rarely. Of course, Western influence has led to an increase in the addition of garlic and sugar to meals in the East as well. Yet Taoists still refuse to use garlic and onions. Ancient forms of Tibetan and Ayurvedic medicine advise against the use of these foods for many reasons:

- Sugar is released in both garlic and onions, especially when cooked.
- Garlic and onions, especially when raw, make digestion more difficult.
- Adding these ingredients lessens our ability to focus and concentrate.
- These foods are members of the lily family, which is known to alter hormone function and be overly stimulating.
- Garlic is useful as a specific temporary remedy, but it is also a potent poison; using it daily, the body becomes oblivious to its me-

dicinal effects.

• Garlic and onions (as well as chocolate) promote heartburn by weakening the muscle at the base of the esophagus.

Close to where I live in Toronto, there are four restaurants that do not add garlic or onions to their food. When I interviewed one owner/chef in the exclusive Yorkville area, a vegan restaurant called Mela, he said that his main reason for not using garlic is the effect it has on digestion, saying that it causes indigestion. Many people notice a distinct problem when they eat garlic and onions and often develop a sensitivity to them, and sometimes an allergic response.

When I studied Tibetan shamanistic medicine many years ago with a Tibetan monk, garlic and onions were among the main foods my teacher eliminated from my diet. Since then, I have noticed that many disciplines that teach meditation and inner focus (including Bon, Taoism, and some sects of Buddhism) ask that one abstain from eating garlic and onions to enhance focus and reduce overstimulation.

Refined Salt versus Unprocessed Sea Salt

Table salt, or sodium chloride, is refined salt, which has no trace minerals and is made more palatable with the addition of dextrose (a sugar used to stabilize the added iodine), anticaking chemicals, potassium iodide, and aluminum silicate.

Some serious health complications may arise without the essential minerals that have been chemically removed from standard table salt. Magnesium is one of these. Without it, calcium cannot be absorbed by the body. Calcium is needed for strengthening bones, nerves, and the heart, as well as for other organs, muscles,

NOTES

and brain development. Most forms of supplemental calcium on the market are not assimilated well by the body, food sources are best, and silica is a plant-derived calcium alternative that is worth searching for.

Lack of magnesium profoundly affects kidney and gall bladder function, making them more susceptible to the formation of stones. Insufficient magnesium also causes an incessant craving for salt. Most people are magnesium- and often potassium-deficient, and our diet does not supply a sufficient available amount to support body function. Restless leg syndrome and cramps in the legs are often remedied by increasing magnesium and potassium. Muscle strength and stress reduction are supported by magnesium in particular.

Refined sea salt has a fine, white grain. Be aware that most of the sea salt that is sold, even in health food stores, is this highly refined variety and not of much use to your body, as the essential trace minerals have been refined out of it.

Unprocessed sea salt sometimes is grayish in color and is slightly damp. (Celtic sea salt is gray with other varying colors, depending on where it is harvested.) The body craves the trace minerals in this salt to keep our blood and other fluids in the right acid-alkaline balance. Unprocessed sea salt contains many essential minerals and trace elements that are very similar in composition to that of our blood. Its alkalizing quality helps to balance acidic conditions in the body. This mineral combination also helps to alkalize the system when we eat acid-forming foods such as

meat, legumes, and grains. Biologists claim that in order for us to maintain a healthy immune system, we must regularly replenish the naturally occurring trace elements, which are available in unprocessed sea salt. Unprocessed sea salt must not be overused, but the minerals it contains are vital to our health.

The correct amount of trace minerals needed is different for each individual. You will know when you have discovered the right balance for you when your craving for salt disappears. Conditions such as swelling in the extremities will also be relieved, blood pressure will level, and you will feel more consistently energetic. The minerals in unrefined salt will also support your digestive system.

Most canned, packaged, and prepared food contains too much processed salt, so read package labels before buying. Part of the effectiveness of the Plan is staying with unprocessed, preservative-free, and hormone-free organic food.

Highly bioavailable (i.e., easily assimilated) trace minerals, as well as sodium and magnesium, are found in sea vegetables such as kombu, nori, dulse, and kelp. Sea vegetables are prominent in the Japanese diet, and they make tasty additions to soups and marinades.

In recent years, people have been avoiding all salt because they are worried about high blood pressure, and since added iodine is the only source of this mineral in many parts of North America, some people are becoming iodine-deficient. Unrefined sea salt contains iodine and magnesium, another mineral many people are deficient in. You can also find sources on the Internet for iodine tests, and powdered magnesium is available at most health food stores. Please refer to the Resources section for sources of unprocessed, trace mineral–rich sea salt, as well as iodine and magnesium.

Additives are Poisons

Conditions such as ADD, ADHD, hyperactivity, adrenal distress, and aberrant behaviors resulting from anxiety and depression are often exacerbated by food additives, colorings, and preservatives. In addition to altering our personalities, these food additives cause the body to retain fluid remaining in the fat cells, causing weight loss to be more difficult. If you don't know the name of what you see on a jar or package label, don't buy it—chances are it has chemical additives that will cause you trouble. In this area it is necessary that you educate yourself and stay aware of everything you put in your or your children's mouths.

Shopping for Sugar

Sugar is in everything. Most of the time I shop at farmers' markets and natural food stores. But sometimes I take myself shopping in supermarkets just to keep current with what else is out there besides real food. What I find always dismays me, but the most recent surprise was sugar in two things I had never thought I'd find it in: olives and pâté. These foods do not need to be sweet!

Over time, we have so corrupted our taste buds that everything must be sweetened or oversalted to have any taste. Because of this addiction to all things sweet, products that don't have sugar just don't have the zing to which we have become accustomed. Our overexposure to table salt, sugar, and preservatives causes

NOTES

food to taste flat and lifeless if it is unsalted or unsweetened. The rapid rise of high blood pressure, heart disease, and diabetes is testament to those deadly taste addictions.

Diabetics have been told that sugar substitutes are fine to use, but recent research has shown that the pancreas responds very similarly to sugar, sugar copycats, and sugar substitutes. This implies that all excessively sweet substances overstimulate the pancreas. The Plan recommends staying away from all sugar and sugar substitutes, other than honey with breakfast in the morning.

What about Other Sweets?

Asparatame is a chemical sugar substitute that is not recommended as a sweetener on or off the Plan. Stevia, a common herb and natural sugar substitute, is regulated as a nutritional supplement, and therefore has more limited access to the market, although it has had more exposure in the last few years.

Stevia is an herb belonging to the sunflower family. Also known as sweetleaf, it is native to South and Central America. Medical research has shown that, unlike sugar, stevia has little effect on blood glucose and it may even enhance glucose tolerance. In addition, research

shows that it may be helpful in treating obesity and high blood pressure.

Xylitol is the newest face on the block of sugar substitutes and has caught up with the pack quickly because it is easily produced—and it has no aftertaste. It also has less of an effect on blood sugar and is absorbed into the bloodstream more slowly. However, it still causes digestive distress for some individuals, so the jury is still out on this one.

After Sugar Addiction Disappears

Stevia in very limited amounts is an acceptable option for later in the Plan, once weight loss has been attained, the pancreas has recovered, and your body has given up being compulsive about sweet tastes. Getting off the addiction to sweet-tasting food, however, is as important in the first stages of the Plan as resolving the problems that sugar and sugar substitutes cause. Doing so allows the taste buds to recover and gives the pancreas a much-needed reprieve.

While off sugar and sugar substitutes on the Plan, you will notice that vegetables begin to taste sweet within a very short time. Your breakfast will be something to look forward to, since it is a full-blown experience of sweet and savory. You will be surprised at the deep

> **Thyroid dysfunction is a very tricky and delicate problem to resolve. Thanks to the Plan, and particularly to Rae Hatherton's wonderful healing skills and advice, I am now able to live a normal life.**
> — *Agathe H.,*
> *Life Coach*
> *Le Châtelet-en-Brie,*
> *France*

sense of satisfaction that just a little breakfast brings.

Hormones: The Controllers

Hormones are the controllers of all major body functions. The most powerful hormones are created and released by the glands of the endocrine system. Of all the hormones, these are the most easily affected by lifestyle, food choices, aberrations in sleep cycles, pharmaceuticals, and stress.

When we put our body in sync with its natural rhythms, hormone imbalances will be corrected. This is a slow process for some people, but worth the effort in the long run. The endocrine hormones are the most finely tuned and most sensitive of all the players in the body's orchestra. When they are working in harmony, the symphony they produce is beyond compare: We are vibrant, our libido

is normal, we are creative and joyful, charismatic and resilient; we are pure power.

Glandulars: The Hormone Replacement Stand-ins

Several medical conditions running rampant in our present-day world are adrenal exhaustion, thyroid hormone imbalance, and pancreatic distress. They can take credit for many of the chronic conditions we are dealing with in our society today. These include anxiety, depression, high blood pressure, digestive problems, addictions, diabetes (high blood sugar), weight gain or loss, and hypoglycemia (low blood sugar). All of these conditions rob us of energy and immune health.

Many symptoms are often caused by adrenal exhaustion alone, including fatigue, low blood pressure, brain fog, inability to exercise, muscle aches and pains, hair loss, eczema, fatty

NOTES

tissue accumulation at the waist, and others. In my practice, I have observed that clients who have adrenal exhaustion also frequently have thyroid dysfunction, and thus impaired metabolism. Thyroid function may be compromised by exposure to fluoride and heavy metals, and since the thyroid is our energy machine, it is difficult to get the fuel burning and the energy pumping in that Maserati with dysfunctional adrenals and thyroid. It would be the equivalent to having the spark plugs and the crankshaft in the engine not working. The car would not run.

Supplementation Is Crucial to Recovery

When hormones are severely out of balance, many people consider supplementing with glandulars, herbs, and/or vitamin-mineral and enzyme support. For individuals whose thyroid is compromised by fluoride exposure or irradiation, herbs are often a solution. Whereas pharmaceuticals may not be subtle enough in their effect, or they may have side effects that many people are not willing to endure, glandulars, herbs, and other supplements can help adjust the release of hormones and assist by supplying more of what the body needs until the affected gland becomes stronger.

Women who have trouble with regulating periods, length and flow of their cycles, or are peri-menopausal (the stage before menopause) or menopausal often have other endocrine organ imbalances.

Glandulars are available in the United States, New Zealand, and the United Kingdom by prescription through alternative health-care providers and in some other countries through a medical doctor trained in alternative medicine. These are powerful substances and are not meant to be used indiscriminately, so it is advisable that you take them while under the care of a professional health-care provider.

Some women with severe hormone imbalance and/or depletion may require compounded hormone supplements, such as "natural" progesterone, estrogens, DHEA, and others that are available by prescription from a physician trained in compounded hormone replacement therapy, and obtained from reputable compounding pharmacies (except in the United States, where some are still available over the counter). The combination of bio-identical hormone replacement, glandulars, and other supplements can restore balance to a severely depleted endocrine system.

I have found that the best results come from consulting a physician who is knowledgeable in this science and who can recommend glandulars, minerals, herbs, and compounded bio-identical hormones produced by a reputable compounding pharmacist. You may need to consult both an MD (allopathic medical doctor) and an ND (naturopathic doctor) unless you are fortunate enough to find a medical doctor with both sets of credentials, or an MD who is self-trained in alternative medicine. Please see the Resources section for alternative doctors and practitioners.

The Supplements

Normal metabolic functioning requires that the following substances be present in sufficient amounts in the body: progesterone, estrogens, testosterone, DHEA, pregnenolone, selenium, iodine, magnesium, calcium, potassium, trace minerals, and the B vitamins, especially B1, B2, B6, and B12.

Nature's Pharmacy

Herbs are part of our natural pharmacy. Nature designed these pharmaceuticals, and we resonate with them—physically, emotionally, and spiritually. Plants are alive; we are alive. Plants vibrate with us and can assist us in healing ourselves. Plants are natural remedies, which, when administered properly, can provide support as the body heals itself.

Unlike drugs, herbs do not take over the function of sick organs. They do not remove bacteria, viruses, and chemical poisons on their own. Instead, they work with the body to stimulate it to help to heal itself. Herbal remedies strengthen the body, helping it to clean its own house and making it more able to defend itself.

Many people who come to the Plan are looking for a lifestyle change that will enhance their quality of life. Many of them are on a pharmaceutical merry-go-round and are experiencing many side effects. Some tell me they just want to get off the merry-go-round.

The herbs used in the Plan have a detoxifying and balancing effect, and thus support our organs and help improve metabolic response, hormone balance, circulation, digestion, elimination, and enzyme function.

For many people, resetting metabolic function with support from natural remedies makes it possible for them to get off their drugs. If you are interested in doing this, you need to elicit the support of your physician before you decrease, and eventually elimi-

NOTES

nate, your prescription drug use. Do not do this on your own!

If your physician is adamantly opposed to helping you, you may want to find a new doctor who is more open to the idea. Your pharmacist may also be helpful in assessing the drugs you are taking and suggesting which ones might not be necessary. Also, you may have some existing conditions that require support, so easing away from prescription drugs may be a long-term, not a short-term, endeavor. Patience and supervision by a health-care professional are required.

Some herbs and natural supplements can conflict with some pharmaceuticals, lessening the drugs' effectiveness, or actually creating adverse effects. If you are taking prescription drugs, it is important that you do not add herbal remedies or teas or nutritional and other supplements while on the Plan without the support of your doctor, pharmacist, and a trained coach (please see the Resources section for trained coaches). In some cases, herbs and supplements can actually enhance the effectiveness of a pharmaceutical, making it more effective, so that less of the drug is required.

The Plan includes an herbal formula, the Cleansing and Transition Tea or Infusion, that assists in detoxification and making the transition to balance. It comes as a loose tea or as an herbal tincture (a liquid infusion preserved in alcohol); both are effective. The herbs in this formula are all safe when used as instructed in the Plan. They are chaste tree berry, sarsaparilla, Irish moss, nettle leaf, parsley leaf, gin-

gerroot, fennel seed, skullcap, passion flower, hawthorne leaf, chickweed, dandelion, schizandra, and cinnamon. The effect of each of these herbs is listed on the product label.

PLEASE NOTE: If you need to continue using certain pharmaceuticals, then these herbs may not be appropriate for you. This does not mean that the program will not work for you, but rather that the effects of the drugs may slow down the progress of the Plan. It is important that you eventually do get off the pharmaceuticals if you want to remedy the condition for which you are using them; however, you must consult with your physician about this and make him or her aware of your wishes. There are some conditions for which you will not be able to stop taking medication. In some cases, if your lifestyle and habits have contributed to the imbalances in your body for which you are being medicated, once you are on the Plan, the conditions may be resolved.

In 2010 Dr. Jamie Nash at the Sullivan University College of Pharmacy in Louisville, Kentucky, set up a pharmaceutical community-support program to help people assess their drug load. (Please see the Resources section.) Many of you may find similar pharmaceutical support networks in your own community. Checking with the pharmacy or medical faculty of your local university is a good start.

Chakras and the Endocrine System

The chakra system used in Eastern cultures,

especially India and Tibet, is a way of thinking of energy and its relationship to the subtle energy systems in the body. It is often represented by a series of wheels at the crown, forehead, throat, heart, solar plexus, navel, and root. Six of the chakras correspond to bodily systems, and the seventh, the crown chakra, is related to all of them.

Tibetan and Ayurvedic medical physiology always includes the chakras as part of the analysis of the body's function. Of course, medical practitioners in the West, even alternative medical practitioners, often think that the chakra system is a bit hokey. There are, however, several medical books that show how the endocrine system and the chakras are tied to each other.

The coauthor (with John Mann) of one of these books, *The Body of Light*, was an old friend and teacher of mine, Lar Short. Lar was the son of a Detroit-born machinist and his wife. One day the couple opened their front door to find a small group of Tibetan lamas on the doorstep. Lar was a reborn teacher, or *tulku*, and the Tibetans had followed the signs of rebirth to his home in Detroit. Lar subsequently passed all the authenticity testing delivered by the lamas. With his mother, Lar was whisked off to Tibet for several years to learn what he needed to become a teacher in the West.

Lar had a unique and wonderful gift of blending East and West from a body-mind perspective. The endocrine system was intimately tied to the chakras in all of his teachings.

The chakras change energy from one level to another by distributing *Ki* (also called *Chi*, *Prana*, and *Mana*) to the physical body. This is partly done through the endocrine system, which regulates other systems in the body. Ac-

NOTES

cording to tradition, each chakra also corresponds to one of the major glands in the body.

There are many approaches to the chakras, and it seems everyone has a different opinion about which glands are tied to which chakra. In my experience, even though I admire Lar's work in all aspects, through my own research and working with my clients, I have established a slightly different set of connections. The following graph supports my experience of the relationship between the endocrine and chakra systems:

The root chakra relates to the adrenal glands.
The navel chakra relates to
the ovaries or testicles.
The solar plexus chakra
relates to the pancreas.
The heart chakra relates to the thymus.
The throat chakra
relates to the thyroid gland.
The third eye chakra
relates to the pituitary gland.
The crown chakra relates to the pineal gland.

Physical, emotional, and hormonal problems are often a result of imbalances in the organs associated with the chakras or the energetic pattern of the chakra affecting the related organ.

The tie between the chakras and the endrocrine system is clear. The chakra system is based on energy, Western physiology is based on function, and the endocrine system runs all the energy-producing systems of the body (digestion, elimination, sexual function, reproduction, moods, emotions, pain control, and many others).

Breakfast and "the Boil"

Some of the components of the breakfast and "the boil" came to me through a nutritionist in Switzerland, Dr. Bueshi, who inspired me to design the Plan based on my own knowledge. Dr. Bueshi came from a small town in the Swiss Alps, and I went to him as a patient for a year. He was very strict about his protocol, and although simple, it was very effective at balancing blood sugar and stabilizing the digestive system. As a practitioner, he had researched his protocol in a diabetic hospital in Switzerland and had had wonderful results.

The breakfast and "the boil" are an integral part of the Alive Plan, whereby during four days of each month during the first part of the Plan, you eat a special breakfast and abstain from alcohol, fat, starch, and natural sugars (other than cooked fruit). This is called "the boil" because vegetables and even meat are boiled rather than steamed (Crock-Pots are often used). "The boil" creates a condition called *ketosis*, which gives your body a short-term fat-burning jolt. Alternating between this and a higher-fat diet stimulates metabolism.

The Breakfast

In the Plan, a delicious spread is made by whipping together honey, cultured sweet butter, and cinnamon. The whipping adds oxygen, which increases its digestibility, and the cinnamon is excellent for balancing blood sugar. Slathering this spread on low-gluten or gluten-free toast, as many slices as you like, or adding it to steel-cut oats or other wheat-free/gluten-free, whole-grain hot cereal, makes a nutritious breakfast and provides enough protein and energy to carry you through until lunch. The result is an almost immediate reduction in the inflammatory response in the pancreas, as well as more balanced blood sugar. Within days, sugar cravings disappear, energy bounces back in the morning, and breakfast is something to look forward to in a very special way.

The Components of the Breakfast and Why It Works

Honey

In the ancient past, honey and butter provided an integral dimension to the remedies that nature offered to the shamans of Tibet, and to the local village doctors in the small, isolated villages in rural India. What nature offered was all these people had to work with. Bees provided pollen and honey, and cows and yaks provided rich butter. Herbs and spices were plentiful and their value understood. Cuts, bruises, burns, and ulcers were coated or packed with herbs. Some remedies were made into a paste with ghee (clarified butter), honey, and preserved herbs. Both honey and butter were used for internal and external treatments.

Laden with antioxidants, antibacterial, and rich in healing properties, honey was available wherever the nomadic Tibetans drifted with their herds. In India, honey was used extensively as a foodstuff and as a preservative in the humid heat, as well as an instant source of nourishment without the necessity of cooking or otherwise changing its form.

Modern applications for honey are being scientifically researched in New Zealand. The

NOTES

nectar of honey bees is now being used in a medical environment for the treatment of third-degree burns. Of all the pharmaceuticals in our wonderful modern cornucopia of drugs, nothing has been found to be as effective as honey in healing and regenerating tissue on severely burned human skin.

Butter

For thousands of years, butter has been used by nomadic people all over the world as a remedy for internal and external ailments. In my research, I ran across some information that supports the use of butter in the Plan breakfast. It also explains why many people, after obtaining the results they desired, continue with the breakfast and continue to have such extraordinary anti-inflammatory responses.

My research shows that if you are fortunate enough to be able to obtain raw butter from cows that have been fed only on green grass, you will be able to enjoy the special benefits of this healthful fat. Please see the Resources section for sources of high-vitamin butter oil, made with butter from unpasteurized milk.

Raw butter contains an antistiffness factor called the Wulzen factor, which protects against degenerative arthritis, hardening of the arteries, and cataracts. In his book *Nutrition and Physical Degeneration*, Weston Price describes another factor in raw butter that he called Activator X, which he found helps the body to absorb vitamins A and D.

In addition, butter (especially cultured) contains arachidonic acid, which is vital to cell membranes and is a precursor to important prostagladins, which modulate biochemical activity. Butter also protects against gastrointestinal infections, especially in the very young and the elderly, and it contains an excellent balance of omega-3 and omega-6 fatty acids.

Cinnamon

In addition to being a favorite addition to food in many cultures, cinnamon has healing factors that are being researched by Western medicine. In June 2007, *The American Journal of Clinical Nutrition* published a Swedish study that showed that cinnamon may help you better regulate your blood sugar levels. The research also showed that the cinnamon concoction used as a test substance appeared to slow the movement of food from the stomach into the small intestine. Researchers speculated that the slowing of digestion might, in part, explain why it lowers blood sugar. Other studies suggest that the spice also may improve blood sugar levels by increasing a person's insulin sensitivity (the ability of cells to respond to insulin's signal to move glucose out of the blood).

Another study published in *Diabetes Care* in 2003 showed that people with type 2 diabetes had significantly reduced blood sugar levels after consuming as little as 1 gram (about ½ teaspoon [2.5 mL]) of cinnamon daily for six weeks. It also improved the subjects' blood cholesterol and triglyceride levels—perhaps because insulin plays a key role in regulating fats in the body.

The Breakfast Recipe

The following breakfast recipe is from my cookbook *The Alive Recipe Collection: Sculpting*

Your Body with Food. Except for the four days each month during "the boil," this breakfast is consumed for the rest of the month during the first part of the Plan.

Honey-Cinnamon-Butter Toast
Yield: 1 cup (250 mL) of spread

Cinnamon oils are very concentrated, and coumarin, the active ingredient in cinnamon, can be toxic in high doses—so stick to the recipe no matter how much you love your cinnamon, and your results will be satisfactory.

½ cup (125 mL) organic, unsalted cultured butter (at room temperature)
½ cup (125 mL) raw honey

½ teaspoon (2.5 mL) ground dark cinnamon
Low-gluten or gluten-free bread, sliced (if wheat bread, sprouted grain only; spelt is fine if it agrees with you)

Put the butter, honey, and cinnamon in a small bowl and whip with a fork until smooth. Toast the bread slices and cover generously with the spread. Eat as much as you need to be satisfied, maybe more at the beginning of the Plan. Cover and refrigerate any leftover spread, and whip it with a fork before using again.

Note: Some people with very unstable low blood sugar will find the honey-cinnamon-butter combination too challenging in the beginning (they might feel light-headed or

NOTES

weak). To remedy this, add plain three or four percent butterfat yogurt (or *fromage blanc* if you are in France) to the recipe. Put the yogurt with two parts butter and one part honey in a small bowl and whip with a fork until smooth. Stir in cinnamon to taste. Once your blood sugar starts to balance, you can go for the fifty-fifty mix, as in the original recipe, and omit the yogurt.

"The Boil"

When I was in my late twenties and early thirties, I was a member of a research organization called The Breakthrough Foundation. This company was founded by Werner Erhardt, a personal-growth guru doing research on organization and teamwork. He used Formula One car racing to illustrate his study, since it required a team of people to work efficiently, quickly, and spontaneously to produce a result; that is, to win the race. For the study, Werner had to lose a lot of weight, but not muscle mass, since the body of a car driver has to be just like the car—lean, strong, and resilient.

At the time, the diet recommended by racing car drivers' physicians was boiled turkey. Boiled fruit and vegetables were added from time to time, but basically, it was boiled turkey. The thinking behind eating this particular food was that it was extremely lean and would burn off all the fat and take none of the muscle or strength from the body, and still provide energy. In three months, Werner was a lean, keen, racing machine.

Don't panic. The idea of boiled turkey did not exactly excite me either, but I discovered a combination of the Breakthrough Diet and a little Atkins Diet added in for good measure. My combination resulted in a short-term solution for fat-burning for the Plan: four days of broiled, grilled, or boiled meat, fish, or poultry; boiled vegetables; and for breakfast, boiled fruit with cinnamon (a compote). And it worked!

The Theory

What is the theory behind boiling food? Boiling leaches fat, not only from the food but also from the person eating the boiled food. Boiling is the best cooking method for removing all fat; broiling is the next most effective method. Adding other boiled food, such as a fruit compote, and boiled (not steamed) vegetables causes the body to burn its own excess fat.

The Atkins Connection

Bob and Veronica Atkins were friends of mine. We met at a couples' club in Jamaica in the early nineties, and since Bob and my ex hit it off, and Veronica and I did as well, we hung out for three weeks in the Caribbean and became friends. Whenever my husband and I went to New York City for business, Bob and Veronica invited us to their place on Long Island for the weekend. We went for walks and talked health and healing, money, and politics. Most important, we cooked and ate.

Bob thought I was a pretty cool cookie. Although he was a respected authority in the alternative medical world, as well as being a cardiologist, I argued with him (which no one ever did) about how he put people into ketosis with the Atkins Diet. I always felt that two weeks was too long for someone to be on a heavy burning cycle. The person would crave sugar after ten days and it was too harsh on the system, especially if the individual was not closely supervised. That was my argument, and we bantered back and forth about it from many directions.

To his credit, Bob actually appreciated my point of view, and definitely my verve for standing toe to toe with him. But of course, he had the evidence of his mass success with his clinic and his books. I know, however, that the thought did spark his interest, since we would debate it for hours. Later in his books he had started to make his system less aggressive from the ketosis point of view—interesting. Either he mellowed with age or I had made a difference. Of course, I would like to think the latter. If he were still around, there's no doubt that we would again have some interesting conversations around the Atkins Diet and what has now become the Plan.

Four Days of Fat Burn

"The boil" calls for four days of eating pure protein, vegetables, and fruit with no added fat, sugar, or starch; in fact, with all the fat boiled or broiled off. All food on this part of the Plan is best done in a slow-cooker or

NOTES

boiled in water (and I mean boiled—like the English do—until the veggies are anything but al dente). Meat and fish can also be steamed, broiled, or grilled. On this part of the Plan there is no drinking of alcohol, even though on the rest of the Plan you can have wine or beer with lunch and dinner. Tea, water, or the Cleansing and Transition Tea or herbal teas are fine.

The name "the boil" was coined by my friend Eunice Ray. Eunice has a great following at Arbonne, a Swiss network marketing company for skin-care products that took off in early 2000. Eunice leaped into the Plan right from the beginning, since she had already been reading about similar ideas on food and hormones, and she brought many of her Arbonne girls on board with her.

Eunice did not look forward to the ketosis part of the Plan, since it turned her breakfast from "honey-butter toast" into a much less exciting fruit compote. When she spoke of "the boil," it was always with a bit of a sour face, since it also eliminated her traditional glass of red wine with dinner. But being Eunice, committed to results no matter what, she took the bit in her teeth and made up recipes to make the whole process more appealing. These she shared with her large following of women, who became a whole lot less large with the Plan. The Arbonne girls also became a lot happier and a lot more successful, pleasing Eunice tremendously. Eunice graciously submitted her recipes for my cookbook *The Alive Recipe Collection*.

On the Plan, the four days of no fat, no starch, no sugar, and no alcohol is repeated every three weeks to coax the body into ketosis. Ketosis is the fat-burning cycle of the body. If your breath smells a little funky and your urine has a distinct odor during this time, do not be surprised, it is ketosis. Going back and forth between this four-day regimen and the high-protein, high-fat, high-starch food of the regular Plan gets the metabolic wheels turning.

Svelte and Sexy in Your Clothes

As you get into the Plan, your metabolic machine will start to gear up and you will notice fat disappearing from places it had not disappeared from in the past. Little pouches of old fat (what they call "brown" fat) will start to melt away and your body will begin to take on the shape of a younger person—less lumpy and pudgy. Of course, there will also be a quite dramatic water weight loss during these four days. The ketosis generated with this plan changes the type of fat burned, so you will not lose any muscle tissue (as happens on most diets that deliver quick results). In fact, your muscles will start to have definition you might not have noticed before.

You may also find that although the scales don't show a great loss in weight, your older, smaller clothes will fit in a way that they had not fit before. The fat will be gone. The muscle will have stayed. Your body will weigh more than it did when you fit your "skinny" jeans, but will take up less room.

If your skin gets loose after these sessions of "the boil," don't worry. It will tighten up. Massage, good lotion, dry skin brushing, and time will take care of it.

"The Boil" Regimen

Do your shopping in advance of the four days of this no-fat, no-alcohol, no-starch section of the Plan.

Breakfast:

Boiled Fruit

Yield: 4 servings

3 cups (750 mL) water
2 apple-cinnamon tea bags
2 large Honeycrisp apples, peeled, cored, and chopped
1 large Granny Smith apple, peeled, cored, and chopped
4 Bosc pears, peeled, cored, and chopped
1 cup (250 mL) raspberries
1 tablespoon (15 mL) ground allspice
½ teaspoon (2.5 mL) ground cloves

Pour the water into a medium-size heavy saucepan and bring to a boil over high heat, and then add the tea bags. Add the apples, pears, allspice, and cloves and bring it just to a boil again, and then lower the heat and simmer, stirring frequently, for about 45 minutes, or until the compote thickens.

Variation: You can use other varieties of apples and berries to suit your taste.

Lunch and Dinner:

Lunch and dinner consist of boiled, broiled, or grilled chicken, fish, lamb, beef, or bison (organic or wild) and boiled vegetables (not steamed). You may use recipes from "The Boil" section of the cookbook, and condiments such as herbs, Dijon mustard, and Celtic sea salt may also be used for flavor.

Note: Do not plan to do "the boil" during your monthly cycle; it is too stressful for the body to handle both at once.

NOTES

Detoxifying

CHAPTER SEVEN

Clutter and Your Environment

Life is a reflection of your inner self. Clutter is a way of avoiding yourself and your wonderful clarity of mind.

Choose one small area in your bedroom, bathroom, or bedroom closet such as a drawer or shelf. Clear and clean it thoroughly. While you are clearing, affirm to yourself, "I am clearing all that I do not need out of my life." Notice emotions, thoughts, and memories from the past that occur while you do it. Be aware of the meaning that you give those items and why you have chosen to keep them or get rid of them. Remember the motto, "Use it, love it, or get rid of it."

— Denise Linn, *Soul Coaching*

My daughter had a company called "Girl Friday" in Louisville, Kentucky. It is one of the ways she supported herself through college, and she still does it by request or on contract. (Please see the Resources section under "Organize Your Space.") Arin helps people organize their houses and their spaces. She always ensures that they have a clear purpose for what they want to happen in their life as a result of the reorganization. Arin understands that when you clear space, possibility opens up. I suggest that you do the same. Be clear about your purpose as you clear the clutter in your house, and then watch what shows up.

Pick small areas at a time and clear them methodically; it does not have to be done all at once. Take your time. Each area you declutter will make a difference in how you feel. Try it!

Clean Out Your Kitchen

Planning ahead, preparing, and bringing things to consciousness are important parts of the Plan. When you begin the program, the first significant step is to clean out your kitchen. There is no point in going through all the recipes, making your grocery list, buying all the food, and steeling yourself for what will be a wonderful ride when there is a chocolate bar lurking in the freezer, just in case.

The kitchen is the heart of your house; it is also the heart of the Plan. Since you will be spending more time there, it is important to have your kitchen set up to support you.

Learning to trust yourself is part of the program, as is having a deep sense of self-respect. It is an integral part of the evolution you will go through. Changing your chemistry will change your attitude, but trusting yourself is just as important.

Kitchens are "catch-alls" for all sorts of things, so go through your cupboards with your eyes wide open and get rid of the following:
- All packaged goods, including canned products that you know you will not be using
- All spices and condiments with added garlic, salt, and additives such as MSG
- All wheat products
- All sugar and sugar substitutes
- Pop, soda, and cola products
- Ice cream, candy, nuts, and confectionary
- Distilled alcohol (put it in the back of your bar or pantry to be used only for guests)
- The stashes of chocolate or candy in the back of your cupboard

If your family is not yet participating in the program, put their treats in a special area of the kitchen, one you commit to not going near.

Make sure you have the new condiments and food that you will need close at hand. This will make it easier for the Plan to work for you. Please see the section "Food Lists" for shopping lists. Also refer to my companion cookbook *The Alive Recipe Collection: Sculpting Your Body with Food*. If you aren't one who cooks a lot, the cookbook can be helpful and you might also consider getting together with other people on the Plan to cook with—or maybe learn to cook. A menu planner at the back of the cookbook is also helpful for planning your shopping trips.

What to Do with All the Stuff

I am sure you have a neighbor or friend who would dearly appreciate these food gifts, at least until they notice your remarkable improvements and start asking about how you've done it. Or you could take the unopened cans and packages down to your local mission or soup kitchen, where they will be more than happy to accept them.

Clean Up Your Life!

Although decluttering may not seem as important to you as getting your body into shape, or even altering your mindset, it does play a very important role in your life.

When I was in training to become a seminar leader for a personal-growth organization in the late 1970s, the initial program was very hard. It was called the GSLP (Guest Seminar Leaders Program) and was designed to move you through a lot of change at what often felt like break-neck speed. As a result, of course, I would often get stuck in the mud of my mind, becoming stubborn and resistant to all of the things that I now know how to work with, but that I didn't back then.

When I got completely buried in the details of my life, when my head was fuzzy and it looked as though nothing was working, the instructors' advice was as follows:

• Clean your house
• Clean your car
• Balance your check book
• Keep your word, especially to yourself

By following this advice, I was able to add structure to my life, promoting clarity. There was also an element of safety in being in control of my circumstances—and we all love to feel safe while in a new process. Being able to see clearly is one of the ways I was able to gain control. Cluttered desks and cluttered kitchens do not promote clarity.

So, with a clear intention to move things ahead, get the family involved or take a day off and go for it. Organize and clean.

Mind Manifests

Have respect for your mind; what you put in front of it is what it assumes you want. One of the best things you can do for yourself and your family is to limit your exposure to TV, newspapers, and media of all kinds. Many TV programs have a negative impact and are not worth watching. Sports are often violent, news is depressing, and believe me, if anything is important enough to impact you, you will hear about it from your neighbors and friends. Advertising often seems to take up more time than program content, and now instead of cigarettes and alcohol ads, we have sexy drug enticements filling the commercial breaks. All this negative external input distracts us from what is important—our sense of self, body, and mind. For now, give it a rest.

NOTES

The Cheerleaders

We all have people in our life who support us in whatever we do and who cheer us on as we accomplish our goals. Hold strong with them while in the first stages of the Plan. People who tell you how great you look, how sparkly your eyes have become, and how much more energy you have are the friends you want around you as you begin this change of lifestyle.

You will gain self-respect from within and you will want to be surrounded by those who give you the respect and acknowledgment that you deserve. Interestingly, as you transform, you will find that you attract more and more of these positive, supportive people.

The Saboteurs

You can't afford to let your happiness depend on the behavior of another person.

— Alan Cohen

Many people in your life would rather see you stay in the same box in which they know you. This is familiar and feels safe *to them*. They may be critical of new things and afraid you are doing something wrong. They may be overprotective. These people likely have issues of their own and may find it confrontational or even threatening to see you handle your issues. They may tempt you, try to get you off track, or argue their point of view to distract you from your own commitment, just to make themselves feel more comfortable.

Please stay clear of these people for the first part of the Plan until you see some positive results and feel strengthened in your own way. This does not mean that you don't care about them, just that you must gain some conviction and faith in your results. For the first little while, keep your openly supportive friends around you. Eventually you will be able to inspire all who come into contact with you!

Forgiveness and Gratitude

If you are holding a grudge toward anyone, and especially someone against whom you have held that grudge for a long time, forgive them. Begin by forgiving them in your mind and your heart, and then progress to letting them know. Anger, resentment, and bitterness are toxic emotions to the mind and body; you may notice when you have these emotions that you feel blocked, rigid, and stubborn. You may find the exercise of embracing and letting go in order to forgive to be difficult, but journaling can often help. Writing a letter to the person if you cannot bring yourself to talk to them can be a beginning.

Learn to be grateful for everything. Begin with the little things, such as when you find a parking spot, or when the lineup at the bank is short, and then expand to the greater things, such as your breath, your body, and your family. You can design your own program to develop "an attitude of gratitude."

Detoxing the Body

Do you not know that your body is a temple of the Holy Spirit, who is in you, whom you have received from God? ...

— 1 Cor. 6:19 (New International Version)

Detoxing applies to body, mind, and spirit, all of which exist in the external and internal worlds of the body. The external is the most obvious. To be surrounded by order and structure makes a difference in your level of confidence and validates the fact that the physical universe loves and supports your actions. When you begin opening the doors to the physical body, there is more mystery involved. The body is able to detoxify on its own. It needs only appropriate action to be taken for it to do so. The body needs to take in clean food and water, but it also needs to be able to put the trash out. Dry skin brushing is one of many actions that can support this process.

Dry Skin Brushing

For many years my practice was focused on very sick people, and I still see a number of people with life-threatening illnesses. I have worked with those who had advanced stages of cancer or autoimmune diseases, including AIDS, Parkinson's disease, chronic fatigue, lupus, and multiple sclerosis. Many of these clients were taking heavy doses of pharmaceutical drugs that were extremely toxic. It is essential to cleanse and support the body in getting rid of the toxic waste as efficiently as possible.

One of the best ways to release toxins is through the skin by increasing circulation in the vascular and lymphatic systems with dry skin brushing. The lymphatic system has a crucial connection with the immune system, as it is associated with the spleen, thymus, and bone marrow and it works with the movement of the interstitial fluid in the body. All bodies need to detox, and when you go through a major transition, such as when you start the Plan, it is necessary to support the detoxification process in every way possible.

The heart pumps blood so it circulates throughout the body. Unlike the circulatory system, the lymphatic system does not have an internal pump. Instead, the lymphatic system relies on movement, in the form of physical exercise, and stimulation. Dry skin brushing

NOTES

stimulates the lymphatic system. Metabolic exercise, such as brisk walking and bouncing on a rebounder, are excellent for moving lymph fluid (please see the section "Metabolic Exercises" in Chapter Eight). Since the lymph carries toxic wastes, which include toxins eaten with food or absorbed from the environment, and which are the natural result of the body's metabolic processes, the lymphatic system is a good place to start detoxification from the inside out.

The skin is the largest organ in the body. Because it plays a significant role in detoxification, it is sometimes called the "third kidney." Other organs involved in detoxification are the kidneys, liver, and lungs. Through perspiration, which is generated by movement, toxins move to the surface of the skin, from where they can evaporate.

Antiperspirants and deodorants are particular bugbears of mine. Chemicals in commercial deodorants go directly into the lymphatic nodes in the armpits. For this reason, please consider using aluminum- and chemical-free deodorants.

Toxins also collect under the skin from such common substances as soap, skin cream, and even from synthetic fiber worn next to

I had fibromyalgia for over fifteen years. After starting this plan, I felt a ninety percent reduction of my pain in two days, my abnormal liver enzymes returned to normal in two weeks, my cholesterol decreased, and in nine months I was off two blood pressure medications.
— Lou Ann B., RN Fisherville, Kentucky

the skin. Herbicides and pesticides are often used to treat materials, and new clothing can penetrate through the outer layers of the skin; therefore, it is always advisable to wash new clothes and dry them in the sunlight and open air to reduce chemical exposure. Dry-cleaned clothes should be taken out of the plastic and aired before wearing. All of these toxins can contribute to a variety of skin problems, as well as to other physical conditions.

Dry skin brushing helps your lymphatic system clear out toxins that accumulate in the lymphatic fluid. This simple technique improves circulation in the skin and keeps the pores open, encouraging the discharge of metabolic and chemical wastes, and thus improving your body's ability to combat infection and inflammation. It also helps your skin look and feel healthier and more resilient!

Every year we lose approximately 7.5 pounds (3.5 kg) of skin through sloughing. It is essential to keep the pores open, the sweat glands stimulated, and detox ongoing.

Here are some of the benefits of dry skin brushing:
• Tightens skin and makes it glow

- Helps digestion through blood circulation and oxygenation
- Helps to remove cellulite
- Stimulates blood circulation
- Increases the rate of cell renewal
- Assists the lymphatic system in the clearing of toxic deposits
- Removes dead skin
- Strengthens the immune system
- Improves the exchange of fluid and trace minerals between cells
- Stimulates the endocrine glands to help all the systems in the body perform at peak efficiency

Dry Skin Brushing Technique

- First, buy a natural (nonsynthetic) bristle brush that won't scratch your skin. Buy one that suits you, long-handled or short-handled, so that you can reach all areas of your body.
- Perform the brushing at least once a day *before* showering or bathing. If you brush on wet the skin, it will not have the same effect and it will stretch your skin.
- Always start on the bottom of your feet and brush in small clockwise circles, moving toward your heart. The soles of your feet have nerve endings that affect the whole body.
- After your feet, brush your ankles, calves, and thighs, then across your stomach, chest, and buttocks, and finally, your hands and arms to your shoulders.
- Make circular, counterclockwise strokes on your abdomen and small clockwise circles on the rest of the body.
- Reach around from the sides, waist, and shoulders to get to all areas of your back.
- Brush more lightly over and around your breasts, and do not brush your nipples at all.
- Brush each part of your body several times, vigorously but lightly.
- After brushing, take a warm bath or shower, followed by a cool bath or shower.
- Use good-quality liquid peppermint soap. Peppermint soap is stimulating and naturally antibacterial, antifungal, and antiviral. If it is too drying, use glycerine soap. (Please see the Resources section for sources for soap and brushes.)
- Wash your brush in warm water every month and let it dry before using it again.

NOTES

Movement

CHAPTER EIGHT

Metabolic Exercises

One of the most important factors for regaining complete and efficient metabolic function is heart rate. Each day we must raise our heart rate above normal and break a sweat. It is best if that elevated heart rate continues for at least twelve minutes and is done three to four times a week.

The best time of the day to get the body going and to elevate thyroid function, and thus metabolism, is first thing in the morning before breakfast. Many of us cannot fit that into our schedule, but knowing that this is the best time can give us the motivation to make it a goal to work toward.

I remember back in the early 1980s, there was a program on TV called *:20 Minute Workout*. I used that program for a few years and found it amazingly effective, easy to do, and an efficient use of exercise time, especially at 6:30 or 7:00 in the morning. It gave me time to get my exercise in before getting my daughter up and out to school and myself off to work. It is this kind of little workout that you need to design for yourself.

Alternating speed walking is one exercise that you can learn to easily incorporate into your life. It is done by walking at a normal pace for two thirds of the time and a fast pace for the last third. If done three or four times a week for thirty to forty minutes, this exercise will elevate your heart rate and give you a sustainable, low-impact workout. This type of workout can also be done in a swimming pool.

Jumping on a rebounder, or mini-trampoline, is another form of exercise that will speed up your heart rate. It, too, can be done early in the morning. One of my clients has her mini-trampoline right beside her bed and jumps onto it before she has a chance to think otherwise. In addition to being an excellent exercise that can raise your heart rate, jumping on a rebounder also stimulates lymphatic drainage. Lack of activity breeds a toxic lymphatic system, which causes sluggishness and congestion and compromises the immune system.

In addition to raising the heart rate, strength-and-stretch exercises should be done daily to promote flexibility and strength. My favorite strength-and-stretch exercises are the Five Tibetan Rites exercises.

The Five Tibetan Rites

When I was studying with a Tibetan monk back in the 1980s, one of the things he taught us was a series of twenty-one exercises to do each morning. We did the twenty-one movements for several years. I was thrilled when I found these exercises modified to just five in a book on the Five Tibetan Rites that showed up in the early 1990s.

For many years in my sessions with my clients, I have taught The Five Tibetans, a simple set of exercises. When done correctly and at the right slow pace, they stimulate the endocrine system in a profound way and provide strength and flexibility. Your body becomes more resilient and energy rises with the ritual and then stabilizes. Digestion and assimilation reach optimum effectiveness. These exercises claim to be antiaging, since they increase the effectiveness of the body's organs and systems.

The Five Tibetans are best referred to in a system called T5T (The Five Tibetans), which was recently developed by Carolinda Witt. The first books I had exposure to describing these exercises were written by Paul Kelder; they are briefer and to the point. Carolinda Witt's T5T is more descriptive, and she eases people into the exercises slowly, with proper breathing technique, structural support, and timing. Having been

> **I was diagnosed with gout in my big toe, and after only five days of being on the Plan, the gout was almost nonexistent! I have also lost over eleven pounds and several inches all over my body. I love doing the Tibetan exercises each morning, as well as eating my 'daily bread' with honey and butter.**
> — *Kathy C., Stockbroker Louisville, Kentucky*

a yoga teacher myself, I also have preferences for the way to do The Five Tibetans, without causing undue stress or possible injury, and yet getting the maximum value from the exercises.

I briefly describe the exercises here, but I highly recommend Carolinda's book to gain mastery in The Five Tibetans. (Please see the Bibliography and Resources section.)

Special Caution: Spinning and stretching through the following exercises can aggravate certain health conditions, such as any type of heart problem, multiple sclerosis, Parkinson's disease, severe arthritis of the spine, uncontrolled high blood pressure, a hyperthyroid condition, or vertigo. Problems may arise if you are taking drugs that cause dizziness. Please consult your physician prior to beginning these exercises if you have any difficult health issues or if you have any other concerns.

1. For the first week, and only if you are relatively healthy and fit, do each exercise three times. Build up by one or two repetitions each week, but only if you feel ready to move on. Even three repetitions will have a result.

2. If you have any concerns whatsoever, please consult your physician (individuals on pharmaceutical medications especially take note).

3. If you are considerably overweight, do not do Rites 4 and 5 until you have developed some strength and endurance; meanwhile, do the substitutes for 4 and 5. (Please see Ellen Wood under "Five Tibetan Rites" in the Resources section for her YouTube video.)

4. Do only what you feel comfortable doing. That may be only one of each exercise for the first week. Build up to two of each ex-

NOTES

ercise the second week, three of each exercise the third week, etc., or at a faster pace only if your body does not hurt.

5. If you have not exercised for some time, prepare yourself by walking for a half hour each day if possible. Yoga stretches also will prepare you for the exercises. If you follow the T5T book, you will not need these preliminaries.

6. Do the Five Rites exercises every day. The maximum number of repetitions is twenty-one; doing more is not beneficial. If you must cut your session short, cut it down to three repetitions for that day.

7. For maximum benefit, do the exercises before breakfast.

Rite 1

Stand erect with your arms outstretched parallel to the floor and with your palms facing downward. Your arms should be in line with your shoulders. Pick a spot on the wall the same level as your eyes, and as you spin clockwise, use this point as a reference. Spin slowly in a clockwise direction. When you are finished your repetitions, lower your arms, look down, and breathe deeply into your belly three times.

Rite 2

Lie flat on the floor, face up, with a small towel folded behind your lower back. Extend your arms alongside your body and place the palms of your hands against the floor, fingers together. Raise your legs to a vertical right angle, hips slightly raised, and at the same time bring your head up so that your chin is tucked to-

ward your chest. Keep your knees straight if possible. Lower your legs and head once again to the floor. Breathe in through your nose as you lift, and breathe out through your nose as you come down. When your repetitions are complete, stay in the same position and do three deep belly breaths.

Rite 3

Kneel on a folded towel with your body erect. Place your hands on the back of your thighs. Curl your toes under. Inhale and let your chin lift slightly as you arch your back. Exhale as you come back to your original position. Breathe in as you stretch back, and breathe out as you return to your starting position. After you finish doing your repetitions, do belly breathing three times.

Rite 4

Sit on the floor with your legs straight out in front of you. Your legs should be extended hip width apart. Put your hands on the floor beside your hips. Slide your feet up toward your hips and lift your body into a bridge until your knees are bent and your calves are at right angles to the floor. Bring your body back down using your legs as support and slide your buttocks back down between your hands. Breathe in as you rise up; breathe out as you come down to your original position. Keep your neck relaxed. After completing your repetitions, do three deep belly breaths.

Note: If you have shoulder problems or are 25 pounds (11.5 kg) over your average recommended body weight, lie down flat on the floor, bend your knees, and lift your torso, keeping your shoulders, arms, hands, and feet on the floor, lifting your body slowly until the middle of your body is raised. Ease your body down, beginning with your shoulders, then your upper back, lower back, and hips. Keep your knees bent and feet flat on the floor. Inhale on the way up and exhale on the way down. Take a breath between repetitions and three deep breaths at the end of the exercise.

Rite 5

Begin this exercise on your hands and knees with your toes curled under. Your feet should be shoulder width apart. Breathe in and raise your buttocks in the air, straightening your legs, and put your weight back onto your hips and feet. Gradually dip down, keeping your arms straight, lowering your hips and moving forward, lowering your body to the floor, arching your back, and relaxing your hips. (In yoga, this is called the upward dog and the downward dog.) Breathe out as you dip down and breathe in as you move your body up and back. When complete, do three deep belly breaths. There are several YouTube videos on the Web, and I will be making one as well.

Tibetan Acupressure

Acupressure is a safe and effective way to move "stuck" energy in the body and to assist struggling organs in an effective and easily maintainable way.

The Tibetan Acupressure System is one that I have developed in collaboration with two Toronto practitioners: a Vita-Flex teacher, Annie Dugan (now retired), and a reflexologist and Nia teacher, Marla Gold. The system is based on a combination of the work of Stanley Burroughs (Vita-Flex), and the original work that I learned from my own Tibetan teacher, Jack.

NOTES

I have since taught the system's mindfulness practice, compassionate touch therapy, and the acupressure points in courses all over the world.

I have incorporated this acupressure system as a part of the Plan to stimulate organ function and to alleviate conditions associated with stress, difficult digestion, and hormone imbalance. It is also useful as an exercise in compassion for oneself.

Often when I work on cancer patients' feet, they have major detox responses; the liver reflex releases, or the head clears, the lymph blockage clears in their legs, or they go home and sleep deeply. Others notice that they feel energized and their body feels light and pain-free.

Tibetan acupressure can be learned easily by the layperson for use on yourself, your family, and friends, and practitioners can become certified in the system so they can add it as a modality to their existing practice. Continuing education courses in Tibetan acupressure can be submitted as credit hours for massage therapy in several countries.

The Tibetan Acupressure System works with the entire body and all its physical and energetic systems. It is a wonderful way to rebalance subtle energies as well as to relax and rejuvenate the mind, body, and spirit. One can sense the body's healing energies realigning. The flow of energy corrects ailments and alleviates and releases tension and stress. The reflexive nature of the system stimulates and settles the system, balancing the body and mind.

These are some of the conditions that can be alleviated or corrected with the system:

- Chronic pain
- Insomnia
- Depression and anxiety
- Mental and emotional stress
- Shoulder and back tension
- Chronic fatigue syndrome
- PMS and menopausal conditions
- Digestive conditions, including reflux, heartburn, constipation, and IBS
- Environmental allergies
- Fibromyalgia
- Sciatica
- Dizziness/tinnitus/vertigo
- Headaches/migraines
- Circulatory conditions, heart distress, blood pressure problems
- Vasculitis and edema
- Cancer (supports immune response and reduces localized pain)

The diagram opposite shows the acupressure points on the feet with their corresponding body systems. You can use the diagram to learn to work on yourself and others to stimulate balanced digestive, elimination, and endocrine functions. The system maps areas and organs of the body on the soles of the feet. Points for the feet and legs generate the most powerful responses, and are easy for individuals to use to treat themselves. A good time to work on yourself is after a meal or in the evening before bed.

Look at this diagram as though you were looking through your feet from the top through to the bottom, as if you had x-ray

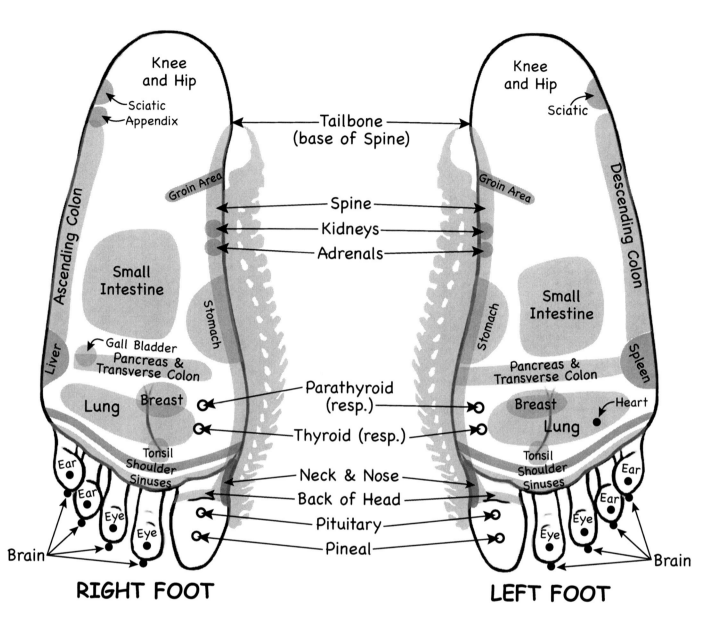

Tibetan Acupressure Points

Courtesy of the Tibetan Acupressure System, © TAS

NOTES

eyes. If you place the diagram beside you while seated and working on yourself, or on a small stool placed in front of your subject, you will have a better idea of how to work.

The system is delivered using the index finger and middle finger of each hand, and sometimes the thumb. The points are touched briefly and deeply with the finger, and by adding a twist of the wrist, the reflex point is deepened. The ankle of the foot being treated is supported with the other hand. There is no stress involved, and movement of the entire hand is incorporated as the finger touches the point and the twist deepens the contact.

Begin the treatment sequence with the right foot, and then move over to the left. The energetic reflex points will stimulate the organs and systems in the entire body, and soothing healing energy will begin to flood the entire system.

For further information on mini-courses in the Tibetan Acupressure System, or for practitioner certification courses, please see the Resources section. Also, please see the video demo on the website at www.tibetan-acupressure.com. You can go to YouTube at www.youtube.com/selfcareforthefeet for a video of my protocol for daily self-care for the feet.

NOTES

NOTES

Communication

CHAPTER NINE

Mindfulness

Mindfulness is a state of nonattachment and absence of clinging to thoughts. When in a state of mindfulness, you perceive things deeply. It is deep observation that leads to a sense of certainty, where doubt is not part of the equation. When fully developed, mindfulness manifests itself as the ability to remain fully present in all situations.

Mindfulness is also a state of curiosity, of examining awareness, whereby observation is as much a part of the practice as what is being observed. It neutralizes delusions and defilements in the mind, and ultimately, combined with meditative *equipoise* (a state of balance acquired through practice), brings the mind to a state that is unaffected by the ups and downs of everyday life. Mindfulness results in a peaceful and invulnerable state of mind, completely unaffected by the normal highs and lows of life.

Mindfulness requires that you become fully present in your life. It may mean that you begin by tying your shoes differently and becoming aware of it. If you have always tied your left shoe first and then your right, try switching the order and then consciously switching it back. Just become aware.

Watchful awareness is a step beyond mindfulness, and it more effectively helps you to "be present." Watchful awareness involves mindfully observing your activities and thoughts as they drift in and out of your mind. It is important not to latch onto or to try to avoid the thoughts, and be sure to catch yourself when you drift into some mental activity. I call it going shopping with your mind. When this happens, call yourself back and begin to observe your actions and thoughts again. When you "go shopping in your mind" again, become aware and make a conscious effort to return to watching.

Being present in order to practice meditation requires calm abiding, mindfulness, and watchful awareness. Sogyal Rinpoche, my teacher and author of *The Tibetan Book of Living and Dying*, says that it requires fifty percent calm abiding, twenty-five percent mindfulness, and twenty-five percent watchful awareness.

Okay, That's All Good, but How Does This Apply to the Plan?

How do we eat? Do we sit down with a knife and fork and mindfully and fully enjoy every bite? Do we savor tastes and smells and textures? Do we take a moment to sit back between bites and restfully sip wine? When we are eating our lunch with our family in front of the TV, at our desk at the office, or in the car on the way to our next appointment, are we being mindful?

Mindfulness and being fully present is what is required to not only enjoy our food but also to have the flavors blend in our mouth with the wonderful enzymes that help make our food assimilate into the next stage of digestion. It is mindfulness that allows the stages of digestion to progress naturally and without effort. Mindful eating may be the best

and one of the most life-giving applications of mindfulness practice.

Eating mindfully has the beneficial side effect of leaving you feeling satisfied, even when you eat less food. How cool!

Exercise in Mindfulness

In today's fast-paced world, we run mainly on automatic and are hardly present in where we go, how we get there, what we eat, and what anyone else around us is doing. In fact, the closest thing we get to mindfulness and meditation is probably TV. At least it has our attention, even though we may be involved in a totally disconnected conversation inside our head while the TV is blaring. Where is the world, the sun, the sky, the wind, or the rose blooming in the side garden?

Multitasking is way overrated. It is the direct opposite of mindfulness, and I attribute much of our ADD (attention deficit disorder) problems, whatever our age, to our living up to this highly touted, but distorted, ideal. Driving the kids to school while drinking our breakfast or listening to the news on the radio, and sitting in early-morning traffic while thinking about our first morning appointment do not demonstrate mindful awareness. And we wonder where the epidemic of adrenal exhaustion comes from?

Perhaps one morning we could let go of a few of the tasks and drive our kids to school without the radio on, without the smoothie, without the mental agenda, just drive and commune with our kids, paying attention to what they ask and what they say. Give it a go! Each of you has your own private version of this scenario, just replace it with your own variation.

HeartMath

Several years ago I was introduced to a wonderful system for maintaining mindful awareness through a program of training in biofeedback that has been extremely effective for people in both their private and their professional lives. HeartMath is a biofeedback technology, whereby the practitioner asks questions while the client is hooked up to a computerized device that monitors pulse responses. The system trains you to notice what upsets you and how to breathe and center yourself through that upset. Through breath and mindful awareness, stability is maintained, and as a result, the pulse rate varies less, the heart rate remains stable, anxiety does not show up, and you feel calm, centered, clear-headed, and in control.

The technology teaches you to use practical interventions such as deep breathing to enable you to reduce stress and emotional turmoil, while enhancing your health, personal effectiveness, and quality of life. Such interventions can do the following:

• Reverse the negative impacts of stress
• Make you feel better more often
• Boost your performance
• Help you find more work-life balance
• Enhance your creativity and decision-making abilities
• Help you overcome chronic anxiety and nervous tension

Please see the Resources section for Heart-Math technology and practitioners.

NOTES

Loving Kindness

Where there is love, do what you will, it will be right action.

— Jiddu Krishnamurti,
Indian Philosopher (1895–1986)

To participate in the restructuring of ideas, and to manifest them physically into new, supportive mind and body habits, you need to adopt and apply the principle of loving kindness toward yourself. In fact, it is impossible to implement the Plan into your life and have it work without applying this practice. Without it, the Plan will become just another diet, a food-oriented, jack-me-up and let-me-down self-sabotage period of life.

Pema Chödrön, the abbot of Gampo Abbey in Cape Breton, Nova Scotia, has a wonderful way of describing the practice of loving kindness. She says it is developing unconditional friendliness toward oneself, feeling at home with our own mind and body, and not looking outside for happiness. It is the realization that compassion and love for others are based on our own happiness and well-being.

The object of the practice of loving kindness is to develop love without attachment and with true compassionate intent. Traditionally, the practice begins with cultivating loving kindness toward yourself, then your loved ones, friends, teachers, strangers, enemies, and finally, toward all living beings.

How does this practice integrate into a lifestyle change? In order to take the time and effort required to change your habits, you need to care enough about yourself to do that, with love. Otherwise, although you will have great results while on the Plan, you will feel and think positively for only as long as you can measure it in weight or feel-good vibes. Then, the minute the speed of the weight loss slows, or you have a bad day, or you forget to breathe or do your exercises, you will find yourself filling the hole of guilt or fear of failure in your heart, your head, or your stomach—the same practice that got you overweight or unhealthy to begin with: lack of self-love. Most of us are all too familiar with this abstain/binge/beat-yourself-up syndrome that often accompanies the effort of changing habits or losing weight.

Participating in this lifestyle requires you to be attentive, mindful, and kind toward yourself. Learning to listen is part of that attentiveness, and developing loving kindness toward oneself is one of the ways of cultivating your listening skills. It is a "being present to what is going on in both body and mind and learning to observe (and not judge)" kind of listening.

In this skill set, there is no judgment, no criticism, no right or wrong. Rather, it is opening up to allow the wee small voice in the body and the mind—the essential self—to be heard and to take its rightful place in your day-to-day living and consciousness.

It is also the skill of learning to distinguish which of the many insistent voices inside is actually the one that loves and supports you, no matter what. That is the voice of loving kindness, not the saboteur's, the internal parent's, or the recalcitrant child's voice.

In our culture we tend to be critical, judgmental, and sometimes caustically cruel in our self-assessment. This type of self-criticism and lack of self-love is definitely part of the human condition.

Many people today live in constant fear of not being loved or lovable. As a result they are starving for approval, from themselves and from others. This can lead to disorders such as anorexia and bulimia, as well as damaging behaviors such as cutting and self-mutilation, or compulsive exercising, studying, or working. Others act out their fears through anger, excessive promiscuity, substance abuse, and antisocial behavior, striking out in the opposite direction as a demonstration of their own lack of self-love.

Some individuals are compulsive about success, others about failure. These demonstrations of the absence of self-love come from externalizing fear and anger. Being aware of this behavior has the potential to develop into what could be a strong sense of self-love. Even in the slickest self-help, self-esteem, and motivational courses out there today, the starting point is still the fixing of a brokenness of the self, followed by actions to make it better—or at least cover up the damage with actions that promise to lessen self-doubt or remove it from conscious thinking altogether.

For the past few years I have added the following quotation by Buddha to the end of every Internet communication I send out. It is meant to remind me that I, and each person I come into contact with, have the possibility to glimpse our true nature in every interaction of life: "Like the moon, come out from behind the clouds. Shine."

So, like the moon, the clouds can part and we can experience our true nature of perfec-

NOTES

tion. It is there all the time. We just need to trust it, to give up the doubt and know it is there. We do not have to cover up our perceived insufficiency, but just know that above the clouds of self-doubt, we are always there, always as we truly are, like the moon in the clear, dark sky, peeking out from behind the clouds.

A Practice of Loving Kindness

Those who cultivate loving kindness toward themselves are, over time, at ease, because they have no need to harbor ill will or hostility. The exercises described below are recommended not only to help you develop self-love and love toward all others but also to be used as an antidote to anxiety, insomnia, and nightmares, since the practice involves relaxing the mind, breathing, visualizing, and creating the experience of thoughtfulness and kindness.

When you work to change habits, you may find yourself being judgmental. This practice opens the way to hearing critical and judgmental thoughts and allowing them to be, not resisting them or believing or grasping onto them. During times of distress and distraction, this practice is a way to provide gentle focus through breathing and mindful awareness that can often completely dissipate emotional turmoil. Have your thoughts, emotions, and sensations. Notice them, observe them, and don't let them have you.

People often notice that when they are around a person who practices loving kindness, they feel more comfortable and happy. It is said that the mind can focus on only one feeling at a time, that when an individual is working toward being kind, it is difficult to become upset and angry. This type of meditation is considered a good way to calm down a distraught mind. Someone who has worked

> **"The Plan cleared my mind and made me acknowledge and challenge the confusion that had been clouding my better judgment and running my life—until now. I realized that the 'magic bullet,' in any aspect of life, does not exist, plain and simple. The minute I stopped searching for it, the noise around me was silenced and the cycle of regret, dissatisfaction, and disappointment came to a screeching halt once and for all."**
>
> — *Danny F.,*
> *Advertising Executive*
> *London, UK*

with this practice will not be easily angered and can, with practice and time, subdue any angry feelings that may arise and make them dissipate.

This practice contributes to one's being more caring, more loving, and more likely to love oneself and others unconditionally. Wouldn't it be wonderful if everyone did this practice? It would truly help us create a world of greater peace, happiness, and inner contentment.

Above all else, we need to nourish our true self—what we can call our essential nature. We so often make the fatal mistake of identifying with our confusion, and then using it to judge and condemn ourselves, feeding the lack of self-love that so many of us suffer from. It is vital to refrain from the temptation to judge ourselves, to lighten up and find the humor in our condition. We need to realize that, at any given moment, others are experiencing exactly what we are experiencing—negative or positive. Having compassion and understanding for ourselves can often open our hearts.

From one perspective, it can be very encouraging to accept that we all have huge problems. It can be even more comforting to realize that in accepting our own pain, we may then be open to be there for someone else. At the same time, it can be comforting to know our problems are ultimately not so real or so solid, or that they are not as insurmountable as we have told ourselves.

Loving Self and Others: An Exercise

1. Sit quietly and comfortably in a supportive chair with your feet on the floor and your hands on your knees, or if you wish, sit on the floor with your legs crossed, back straight, and shoulders relaxed.

NOTES

2. Gently breathe into your belly through your nose, and out through your mouth very slowly. Settle, take your time, and relax. Do this several times.

3. Find, from your present or past, someone you love. If that is too difficult, remember some music you love or a favorite pet, a painting, or a wonderful view.

4. Then remember someone who loved you: an adult, a baby, a child, or even a dog or cat, and remember what it felt like to bask in their love. Just recall what it felt like to be loved. Allow those experiences of loving and being loved to permeate your body and mind.

5. Next, remember someone who is very dear to you, a daughter or son, a spouse, a mother or father, or dear close friend. Send the experience of love you have just found in yourself out to them. Then think of someone else you love and send the feeling of love out to them. Continue this process, being very patient with yourself until you cannot think of anyone else to whom you would like to send out love. Note: if you have trouble with this part, remember this quote, which Pema Chödrön attributed to her teacher: "Everybody loves something, even if it is only tortillas." Just remember the feeling of love and extend it out.

6. Begin to keep the following lists. Take your time and keep adding to your lists. You may want to keep them on your computer or write them in a small book so that you can continually add to them as you live your life.

i. Make a list of all the people and animals you care about and are close to and repeat steps 1 through 5 and send love out to them. Remember your own heartfelt experience of loving and being loved every time.

ii. Make a list of people who you know as friends or acquaintances, touch into your love, and send it out to them, one by one.

iii. Make a list of all the people you don't know: the politicians, people in third-world countries, people just like you elsewhere in the world. Remember your love and send it out to them.

iv. Make a list of people who feel animosity toward you or who you regard as your enemies. Remember your love and send it out to them.

Take your time and add to your list as you feel ready. At first you may be able to send out love only to the ones you are close to, and it may be a long time before you are able to move on. That is fine; take it slowly if you need to.

Practicing loving yourself and others will set the tone for your day. It will only take a few minutes and a few breaths, and it will help you to be genuinely present for yourself and others in day-to-day situations. You may find that you need to do this breathing practice often as you go through your day, forgiving yourself and remembering to love yourself rather than berating yourself for a decision or a comment. Ease yourself into having permission to make mistakes, replacing justification, defense, or anger toward yourself. And take your time. Be patient. You will actually become more successful and content as you progress.

Rewarding Ourselves with Damage

For some reason, and I have yet to discover how or when this happens, we reward ourselves with harmful indulgences. Have you ever noticed that you often celebrate in unhealthful ways, and that it can sometimes cause serious damage?

We go out drinking to celebrate a victory after a ball game. We have huge cakes at all special events like weddings and birthdays. We have gross volumes of food on holidays.

We reward ourselves for work well done with a cigarette, a cigar, a chocolate bar, or a big meal.

Why is this? Why don't we reward ourselves with a massage, a pedicure, a walk in the park, or a meditation session? Why do these types of activities not have the same level of satisfaction?

Addiction is one of the reasons. We are addicted to stimulants and overindulgence, and we use the occasion as an excuse to indulge. Bringing these kinds of actions to conscious awareness is the first step toward stopping the unsupportive action. When you have inclinations toward rewards that are harmful, try to catch yourself and switch to a reward that is supportive of your well-being.

NOTES

Meditation

All of our auditory and visual diversions—movies, television, radio, cell phones, iPods, email, instant messages, chat rooms, games, sports, and whatever else you're into—these are all mental diversions designed to keep us from discovering our own inner voice.

— Alice Ruddy

Many of my clients have severe adrenal fatigue. Much of this fatigue comes from the constant input of technology and media. The pace at which we drive ourselves doesn't help either. Seldom do individuals nowadays take time to lay back and look at the clouds, or to just sit quietly for an hour without stimulation of any kind. The breakdown of the adrenal glands is a sign of overload that can affect many other organs of the body and begin a cascade of symptoms, thereby resulting in disease states of all kinds. Sitting down in daily contemplative meditation is a way to settle the adrenal response mechanism.

Meditation is called the Great Teacher. It is the cleansing crucible fire that works slowly through understanding. The greater your understanding, the more flexible and tolerant you can be. The greater your understanding, the more compassionate you can be. You become like a perfect parent or an ideal teacher. You are ready to forgive and forget. You feel love towards others because you understand them. And you understand others because you have understood yourself. You have looked deeply inside and seen self-delusion and your own human failings. You have seen your own humanity and learned to forgive and to love. When you have learned compassion for yourself, compassion for others is automatic. An accomplished meditator has achieved a profound understanding of life, and he inevitably relates to the world with a deep and uncritical love. Meditation is intended to purify the mind. It cleanses the thought process of what can be called psychic irritants, things like greed, hatred and jealousy, things that keep you snarled up in emotional bondage. It brings the mind to a state of tranquility and awareness, a state of concentration and insight.

— Bhante Henepola Gunaratana, *Mindfulness in Plain English*

Meditation is a badly misunderstood skill. You would think that with all of the successful meditators out there, the information for the public would have become more accurate. What I always hear from my clients, friends, and students is, "Well I tried it but I just couldn't still my mind." For some reason people have the idea that they must still their mind to be successful at meditation. Not so; in fact, if you could continually still your mind while meditating, you wouldn't need to meditate.

The function of the mind is to have thoughts. That is its job. Your function as a person meditating is to get enough distance from your mind to watch those thoughts, not be them, not act them out, just to have them. The real point is to have your thoughts and not to have them have you. If you need motivation, remember that the greatest gift you can give yourself or anyone else is full, unconditional presence. It is what everyone needs; it is the highest expression of love. The only way I have found to get oneself out of the way enough to become that fully present is through meditation.

All meditation requires is that you take some time every day in a quiet place—with your cell phone turned off. Sit up with your spine straight, shoulders and neck relaxed, your eyes open and looking slightly down so that they are relaxed. Sit quietly and focus. It often helps to have something to gaze upon, such as a flower, a candle, or an inspiring pic-

ture of nature or a deity. (If you are sitting in a place such as a park, it can be a blade of grass, or if in a railway station, a pattern on the floor.) Position the object a short distance in front of you so that your gaze falls upon it in a relaxed manner. When you get distracted, catch yourself gently, come back to focus, and begin to be present again. Just watch your thoughts go by; let them go as though they were separate from you and floating. Bringing your awareness to your breathing can also help to bring you back to being present, focused, and relaxed.

Take your time, take frequent breaks at first, just shake yourself, take a few deep breaths, a sip of water, and go back to sitting.

Meditation from another Point of View

In all my work counseling and teaching peo-

NOTES

ple, I have always tried to bring meditation into their lives. There are many different kinds of meditation, and over the years I have learned many of them so that I would be able to share my knowledge with others. However, I have found that often people don't feel that they have the patience or the discipline that meditation requires. Perhaps one percent of the people I have worked with really take to meditation practice and hang in with it.

Some people have trouble just sitting for any length of time without something to listen to. If you have this problem, I recommend a CD called *Holosync*, produced by the Centerpointe Research Institute (please see the Resources section). Holosync is a brain-balancing meditation CD of nature

> **Within three months I saw fairly significant changes in my nervous system. I work in live TV and found that I no longer got nervous during any of our shoots. Ever. And that calm sense of well-being I had went with me everywhere I went. Meeting new people? A breeze.**
> **I could even remember their names, and it was so natural now for me to stay in the moment of our conversation, rather than be thinking ahead. Staying in that moment made these conversations so much more valuable, and also made the people I was talking to feel that I was actually listening. And I was.**
> — *Donna BB., TV Sports Anchor*
> *Louisville, Kentucky*

sounds. You begin by listening for a half hour a day and then progress to an hour. *Holosync* "meditates you"; in other words, it does the work, and you just need to sit there.

In the 1970s I used subliminal tapes as a way to help me become calm and happier, and to get the benefits of meditation without as much effort. Regrettably, the quality of the tapes was not that good, as the technology was still in its infancy, so the results were proportionate.

Since that time, the brain—its frequencies and its effect on human physiology and psychology—has been the subject of many scientific studies. Research has allowed for new and improved technologies for bringing brain frequencies into balance.

These advances have resulted in tools that enhance performance and mental acuity, increase happiness and feelings of peace, and provide many other benefits. Please see the Resources section and the Bibliography for tools and literature on meditation.

All We Really Want

All we really want as human beings, every single one of us, is peace and happiness. We go about getting peace and happiness by trying to arrange our circumstances, such as making money, getting married, having a good job, and doing all that our culture and society tells us will give us happiness. But it never works. Actually, it does work for a moment, a day, a week, or a few years, but it doesn't last.

There are two qualities of mind, one is that of appearance and the other that of essence.

The acquisition of things and attaining a quality of life in the outer world bring interim contentment. That interim contentment is temporary and is a function of the ordinary mind or the mind concerned with appearance.

The quality of mind that works with mind's essential nature, which involves meditative *equipoise* (a state of balance acquired through practice), is what brings one to a state of inner peace and contentment that cannot be shaken and that no change in circumstance will alter. This is the essence of mind that we truly long for to connect us to the kind of fulfillment and contentment that is long-lasting and what we truly long for.

Time spent daily is what is required, so even a few minutes are better than not at all. Sitting on an airplane or in the bathroom can

NOTES

be your time; take it, and eventually it will become so important to your quality of life that you will make time for it.

Over time, as you settle into the meditative technique, whether a simple practice of sitting looking at a candle, watching the breath, or using *Holosync*, it is necessary to get to the point where you do not need support from a CD or an object to focus on. This is the goal to work toward, but not to demand of yourself. The effort applied in just sitting quietly will bring wonderful rewards.

Learning to Listen to Your Body: The Door to a Balanced Life

One of the most important skills you will learn on the Plan is how to listen to your body. We live in a culture that is based on external input. We are bombarded by various media with visual, auditory, and sensory data every day, yet we seldom listen to our body's response to this onslaught. We are addicted to and hypnotized by the external stimulants of sugar, pharmaceuticals, chemicals that are added to our food and drink, and noise, all of which make us numb to the internal dimensions of our mind and body. Worry, financial concerns, looking good, dressing attractively, and staying current with trends in cars, clothes, and news have become so important that we have neglected true values.

The Alive Plan will open the doors to finding balance. Life may not slow down, but it will feel more paced. You will relax into the structure of three meals a day, sleeping at times that work, and keeping extremes out of your lifestyle. Eating good, fresh food and experiencing good digestion and elimination, breathing fully, and exercising will give you stability. You might be surprised at the sense of safety that creeps into your experience of this fear-laden social environment in which we live. Structure offers safety—security in a familiar sense of order. All living beings thrive on order, and as so, so do we.

Listening to your body means learning to tabulate its response to food and other input. Your body always knows what works and what does not, and you can feel it when you pay attention. The neat thing about learning to listen is that once you start, your body will take the cue and let you know what is going on loudly and clearly. Once you open the door to trusting your body's voice, it will let you know what works and what does not.

One of my clients told me that she was feeling so fabulous on the Plan, losing weight, looking good, sleeping well, and for the first time in years, getting off antidepressants and adult ADD pharmaceuticals—she was on five drugs in total! But one day she had a piece of cake and promptly fell very ill. Her body had given her a message: "Don't do this to me now, you have been so kind, and now this?" Lisa returned to the Plan immediately, but only after she had related her experience to all her friends via the Internet, letting them know that she got the message.

Perhaps if we learn to listen to our body and our own inner guidance with thoughtful attention, we, too, will be able to be present for and listen to others.

NOTES

Support

L iving the life of your dreams is a lot like sailing. You pick your destination, hoist up your sail, make minor adjustments while the journey is underway, and let the wind do all the hard work. In other words, imagine the end result, do what little you can, make minor adjustments while the journey is underway, and let me blow your mind. Phe-e-e-e-e-e-w!
— Mike Dooley, *Notes from the Universe*

Support on the Plan means having people, activities, and techniques that help you make the transition through the first stages of the Plan effectively and with ease. I have already discussed the kinds of support you can give yourself: being mindful, learning to practice loving kindness, listening to your body, and practicing mindfulness and meditation.

You have also learned about how to detoxify your external and internal environments, and you have been given guidelines to help you get through the rough spots as you make the lifestyle changes that will help you reach your long-term goals. I also discussed the exercises and bodywork that you can use to ease your body more gently through the shifts you will experience as the Plan becomes an integral part of your life. And now, in this chapter, you will learn about the importance of the outside support you can get from friends, family, buddies, and coaches that will really make the difference as you change your life.

Partners on the Way

Support is an intrinsic part of what makes life work. Without support, I could not have written this book. There are so many people who appreciate what I have been doing with the Plan and understand how it benefits others. These people have offered their support by sharing their experiences on the Plan, holding support events for friends in their homes, enrolling others, offering to type and edit, and setting up and running my appointment schedule in the towns where I have speaking engagements. There are so many different towns and cities in which the Plan has come to be a household word, and this support has been critical in allowing me to coach so extensively. All of this assistance emanates from a desire to see others healthy and to support a vision of a healthy community.

Just as I could not have written this book without support, I suggest that you will find staying with this lifestyle much more a labor of love if you have support from other people, and if you support others. Find yourself a buddy or a group of people to partner with on the road to a lifestyle of health and well-being. Hopefully, it makes the road smoother and definitely more fun. Make sure the person or people are committed to change no matter what, just like you!

Motivation

Support also works because it keeps you motivated. The support from those people who have achieved health and happiness on the Plan can only inspire and motivate those who are just beginning. And when we achieve our goals, it is natural to want to support and assist others in turn. Not only that, but seeing the success of those we support can inspire us anew. Help and support are invaluable because this regimen is not always an easy path to take, and the vision can sometimes seem elusive.

There are barriers and hurdles, slippery slopes and discouraging situations. Rough patches occur when you decide to change your metabolism and your lifestyle and begin to move your life in the direction you always wanted. Encouragement can make all the difference to your success.

The Buddy System

The true way to soften one's troubles is to solace those of others.
— Madame de Maintenon (1635–1719)

Having a buddy to share in your journey will help you, especially during the first stage of this program. Many people have no problem being disciplined and can follow along from one appointment (if they are being coached) to the next with no sidetracking. For others, it can prove to be more difficult. Having a friend as a supportive partner or a spouse who is willing to go along this path with you makes the journey that much more enjoyable.

Another kind of buddy is someone you would like to support and bring along with you on the journey. It may be best to wait until you have some results under your belt, and then share those results with someone who needs your support. This will also inspire you to inspire them.

You can also continue to be inspired by staying in touch with the network of support that you'll have through the website, along with our email support and telephone appointments (if requested). Eventually, a time will come when you feel strong enough to use your newly developed communication skills to gently address those individuals who may feel insecure about your great results.

The Plan often has a life of its own. One of my many clients who has had success with this lifestyle change and has gone on to support others is Martha, who became one of my superstars. She completely renovated her looks, her energy, and her life. A manufacturer's rep in the furniture industry, she just walks into her clients' stores and they are all over her, asking what she has done to account for the dramatic change. As a result, she has her own following of people, and since these people are her clients and she is in touch with them regularly in person, by phone, and by email, she can support them, and she is just as thrilled with their results as she is with her own.

Most of us want to have others, as well as ourselves, succeed. Partnership and empowerment are facets that bring joy to life and make the path to success more pleasant, less lonely, and in the long term, more sustainable. Bring along your spouse, your daughter, your best friend, or a group of friends on your journey.

Coaching

When I was young, in fact from as early as I can remember, I was an avid swimmer. It was

NOTES

my passion. When I began to take swimming lessons, even though it would be two years before I was old enough to qualify for all my badges, I took and passed all the tests. I just loved to swim.

When I was eleven years old, I decided to train for a twelve-hour marathon that was being run by our local community center. There were a few of us who were dedicated, physically fit, young swimmers. We took all summer to train, swimming lengths, exercising, and extending our training times as the summer progressed.

My coach and pacer was a wonderful man, whom I admired and respected and who guided me in my training. His name was Alex Vanderzand, and I will never forget his gentle guidance and constant encouragement.

The marathon day came; I was set—trained and ready. The early part of the day was fun—lots of people, noise, and interaction. Things were just swimming along for the first many hours. My training really showed up. Then it all changed. I was into hour ten when I suddenly started to get cramps in my legs. My calves tightened up, I was treading water trying to massage them. I panicked a little with the pain, and my blood sugar levels dropped like a stone. The cramps dissipated and I started to pace myself again, but the damage was done. My body became very cold and I started to fall asleep in the water as I swam. The support team yelled encouragement to me from the sidelines, but it was as though I was on automatic pilot, numbed to the sound, my body was just stroking along. I kept on going in spite of the residual pain in my legs; it seemed as though they were part of someone else's body.

Alex, seeing that I might be in trouble, stripped off his outer clothes, and bearing hot chocolate in a "sippy" bottle, jumped in and started to talk to me quietly as he swam alongside, and gradually I came back to my body. When I was fully back and aware of my body, the pain in my legs, the fatigue, and the shock of having Alex right there made me panic a bit and I went under. Since the rules were that he could not help me except to assist me from the side or provide encouragement in

> **I sleep better and for a shorter period of time. I feel better, I have more energy, I am fun to be around again (and not depressed). I lost weight, and I can think more clearly. I know if I go back to my old ways, my problems can come back. It is great motivation to stick with the Plan.**
> — *Annie H., Licensed Massage Therapist Crestwood, Kentucky*

the water, Alex waited until I surfaced, and then he started talking. He paced my strokes with me and gave me the hot chocolate, and the warmth of it brought me back. It was his support and presence that got me through.

Knowing my nature well, one of the tricks Alex used to get me to the finish line was to dare me to get out and dance the twist on the pool deck when the marathon was over. (It was the coolest dance around then, honest.) Usually, when a marathoner gets out of the water after twelve hours, it is quite difficult to stand, let alone dance, but the thought inspired me and kept me going through the last few grueling hours of swimming. All of that caring and daring gave me the energy that I needed to complete the marathon.

When I stepped from the water to the mu-sic of Fats Domino, I danced with Alex for a few minutes to the cheers of my friends before collapsing. I will never forget having been able to achieve that impossible feat—all made possible with the courage and determination with which Alex had inspired me, right at the moment when I was most ready to quit. His perceptiveness, his good instincts, and my own drive led me to success and beyond. That is a true coach!

A coach is someone who participates with you, trains with you, and stands on the same side of the fence with you. The coach may not have had exactly the same experience as you, but he or she will have compassion for exactly where you are, and will know what to do to support you in your next step toward success.

NOTES

Coaching and the Plan

God, grant me the serenity to accept the things I cannot change, the courage to change the things I can, and the wisdom to know the difference.

— Reinhold Niebuhr,
American Theologian (1892–1971)

Coaching is a crucial part of this lifestyle change. Coaching and partnering with others is the support that gets you through to the next stage. When you run out of steam, get in touch with your coach. When you run across what seems like an insurmountable obstacle, it is the coach who makes a "molehill out of the mountain." It is when you pull that two-by-four out of the closet to beat yourself for something pretty insignificant that your coach makes you laugh at yourself. Your coach will be inspired and moved by your courage, and thus, so will you.

Coaching is a trained skill. It is much better if the person coaching you has been through some of the same things as you, but it is not absolutely necessary. Coaching is as much about listening, providing support, being there, and giving direction as anything else. With the Plan, it is necessary to have a coach who has hung in and had personal accomplishments, even if the area of his or her success is not the same as yours.

Coaching is love in the guise of cheerleading. It is what the sponsors at Alcoholics Anonymous are trained in and what makes Weight Watchers and other support systems like it work. It takes accountability, commitment, inspiration, and courage.

Guides in Life: You Can Do This Program by Yourself, But ...

Without an escort, you're bewildered on a familiar road; don't travel alone on a way you haven't seen at all; don't turn your head away from your guide.

— Rumi, Muslim Poet, Theologian,
Sufi Mystic (1207–1273)

All of my life, I have turned to a guide. I have found guides in every practice and body of learning I have followed, of which there have been many. Learning to surrender to the guide—learning to do what someone who cares enough to tell it to you straight, and to set aside your attitude, ego, and righteousness to do what has been proven to work—is what turns it all around.

I was hesitant about writing this book at first, because I was concerned that I would not be there to answer all your questions, to help you get over your stumbling blocks, and to address your concerns and your changes. Somewhere in the past few years, when I began working more and more by email and by phone, I started to trust the fact that if you really wanted or needed information, guidance, or coaching, you would find me, set up an appointment, and communicate. So here we are. Now I am training others to be there, I have a sincere wish that many people will train as practitioners to be able to be there for people as they transition into this new lifestyle.

Yes, this plan is my program and my system, so I know it better than anyone else. But there are a multitude of resources from which you can get support. Feel free to send me an email, call me, or ask someone who has done the program to contact you. Or, if you'd like, you can set up a personal coaching session. Coaching sessions will always give you exactly what you need at the time you're looking for it.

Making It through Successfully

One coaching session a month in person, by phone, or on Skype is ideal to keep you sailing in the right direction. Sailing offers a great metaphor. Often, although clear about your destination, you must tack (go back and forth to catch the wind), and it may feel as though you are going in the wrong direction for a while. Having someone tell you to tack (adjust direction) when you need to is more than useful. The ship gets back on course that way. Most people who have successfully made it through this program have done it with coaching. Sessions can be conducted by phone or Skype and followed up by email (which is always included as part of the coaching fee).

It takes three months to a year for most people to get through this program (exceptions are those who have over 60 pounds [30 kg] to lose and those who are on more than one prescription drug or have a major immune system illness). In such situations, more time is required.

For more information on coaching, websites, and practitioners, please see the Resources section.

NOTES

ALIVE!
An Energy
Plan for Life

CHAPTER ELEVEN

Guidelines

Now all that is left is for you to become yourself.

— Johann Wolfgang von Goethe,
German Writer (1749–1832)

Structure is vital in life. Without structure we would not be able to function as human beings. When I studied massage therapy, I saw the importance of the skeletal system. It provides a structure in which to house the body's organs and systems, and a frame around which to build muscle, nerves, and tissue. Structure is framing; it sets up a context for things to exist within and work. Structure works within structure; it is a living, evolving framework for life and workability. Our body calls out for external structure to support the internal. Its building blocks are very simple; our body loves simplicity but needs structure.

Many of our traditions, such as eating three meals a day, eating together at supper, working nine to five, and going to church on Sundays, are now almost nonexistent. They have been lost in the aggressive drive for accomplishment and accumulation. In the past, those structures, rituals, and traditions provided a structure of workability, sanity, and a feeling of connectedness that is fast disappearing. Structure gives us a place to live, to function. It provides a sense of trust for what we know works, and within that space creativity and innovation grow. That forms the framework for life.

Structure can also be limiting. We can use it to cage ourselves. It is this kind of structure that I would like to avoid with the Plan. As with anything that works, some discipline is required, although some may think this is limiting. Imposing discipline on oneself with an ultimate goal in mind is not limiting, it just narrows the path and focuses on a direction that, when followed, will produce the desired result. It could be viewed as freedom from what is unworkable.

When you start on the path, it is to discover what works for your body and what does not. The first stages of the Plan have some limitations—lots of structure—and granted, your life will have to change to incorporate them. Many people have said that once they surrendered to the Plan, it was the easiest thing they had ever done, because it made sense—just common, everyday sense—and it felt very ordinary, very easy, very basic. The only thing that was in the way of their doing it from the beginning was their own resistance.

Remember the Borg motto from Star Trek, "Resistance is futile"? Another slogan from my past was, "Whatever you resist persists." Resistance holds things in place, it is a force of nature or the universe, which, when used properly, provides support and, when used with attitude and force (heels dug in), stops progress and inhibits results.

So make things easy for yourself and simply ask: "What by when?" Make a little promise. Eating the elephant in small bites makes it a much less formidable enterprise. Day by day,

commit to one new change, one new habit, one new addition or elimination. You can make each change daily, weekly, or monthly, too; there is no rush. Take your time; add or take away at your leisure. It took you a long time to get where you are, and this is a lifestyle change, not a diet. Not an overnight renovation but a new way to become more *alive*.

Surrender is another word that makes people flinch. It always seems that surrender is mistaken for giving up, abandonment of hope, or yielding. In this case, surrender is just giving up control and allowing a functioning structure to work its magic.

A good question would be, then, "To what am I surrendering?" Are you surrendering to what you are committed to, or to an external expectation, what you want or what someone else expects, including your boss, your spouse, your family, your friends, your teacher, or *Vogue* magazine?

In this plan you are surrendering to your higher aspirations for yourself, who you know you are? Surrender happens from the inside out. So as one teacher of mine, Marshall Thurber, said so eloquently, "Trust the dance."

The Power of Visualization

The mind works in pictures. By visualizing what I want, I get the picture—literally! Create what you want by visualizing it. Put it in front of your mind. Here is a tool you can use as you begin the Plan:

1. Take a photograph of yourself at the beginning of the Plan and put it away. Then

find a picture of yourself that was taken at a time when you felt great and looked great. Put that photo on your refrigerator door. If things are not happening as fast as you would like down the road, pull out that first picture; you will be surprised!

2. Find a pair of pants or a dress that you love, but can no longer fit into. Hang it on the door of your closet. This is meant to inspire you and to show your mind the direction in which you wish to go. Later on, when you finally put on those pants or that dress, you may be surprised that your body is in even better shape than when you last wore that outfit and that it is not as appealing as you anticipated. If this happens, then go out and buy a new outfit!

As you change, change your wardrobe. Get rid of the larger clothes and get new ones—consignment shops are great for the transi-

tions along the way.

I had a pair of Donna Karan jeans that I just loved, and those were the ones I hung on my door. When I finally put them on, my body had changed shape so much (in a good way) that I didn't like the way they looked anymore, and I went out and bought a new, more fashionable pair. One of the things this demonstrated to me was that what I remembered in the past as being exactly what I wanted turned out not to be what I wanted at all.

Keep a Record

If you want or feel you need to keep a journal of your food intake and weight as well as your feelings and sensations. Keeping a record of what you eat helps to keep you conscious and lets you know what is working and what is not for your particular body. Journaling is a wonderful way to acknowledge your progress

NOTES

and allow your insight and feelings to come out in a constructive way. *The Artist's Way* by Julia Cameron is an old standby for learning to journal.

A Word about Scales

Weigh yourself when you start the Plan, if you want to. Be sure to weigh yourself only once every two weeks—no more, and always on the same scale and at the same time of day. It is often a good idea to see how far you have come by seeing it on the scale, and also to notice that your size and shape may have shifted, but sometimes the scale has not. Weighing yourself can help your self-esteem when you feel it is wavering. Trying on clothes is also a good way to support your progress. It is important to remember that this is not a weight plan. You may have lost two clothing sizes and have it show up on the scale as only two or three pounds. Many people have issues with scales, so don't weigh yourself if you are one of them. Your body will "morph" into a new shape, shift, and alter composition, and this can't be measured on a scale.

I have always allowed people, including myself, to do whatever works. Scales usually don't work for me; if my judgments and fears show up, I don't use them. I use measurements and clothing size (clothing I already have).

A useful way to keep track of change so your mind does not trick you into thinking you have made no progress is to keep a record of your measurements. Make sure you measure in exactly the same place every time. As with weighing yourself, do this only once

every two weeks and no more.

Additional Basics

Here are some guidelines for the Plan that are quite vital to its success, especially at the start. The beginning stage sets up your body to start tuning the metabolic process. Each one of the following tips will help speed up the process and make it more effective.

Exceptions for Meals

- If you miss the time allotted for breakfast, wait until lunch for your next meal.
- If you miss the time allotted for lunch, eat in the mid-afternoon, up to 3 p.m.
- If you are late for dinner, eat late and miss eating breakfast the next morning.
- One late dinner is permitted every seven days during the Cleansing and Transition part of the Plan; however, it works best if you skip breakfast if you eat later than 8 p.m.
- One lunch or dinner a week of black tea and heavy cream is permitted (as much as you like), except for those who have blood sugar issues.

Make sure you eat well at meal times. Eat until you feel comfortably full (which you may not be aware of at the beginning, since emotional eating is often the reason for eating more). Learn to listen to what your body is asking for, and what feels comfortable in your stomach. You will be less into "survival," or fear of going without enough, in relation to food as you progress on the Plan and the results start to happen. So relax and enjoy the ride.

Adapting to the Plan

Sluggish systems may take a while to kick in and may need support from supplements. Any kind of change, for some more than others, may cause conditions such as constipation, upset stomach, and change in sleep patterns. Most of these complaints will resolve themselves with a little supplemental support. Add magnesium at night for sleep and elimination support, as well as a liquid trace mineral and iodine to your regular supplement program. Digestive enzymes are useful to help digestion, and added hydrochloric acid and pancreatic enzymes help those with a sluggish digestive system.

Each body is different. Natural thyroid and other hormone supports may be needed. We can advise you or direct you to a practitioner who can assist. You might want to set up a consultation, have a conference with a buddy, have an email support chat, or go to the blog on the website (listed in the Resources section) for specific instructions. Getting some expert advice if you are feeling stuck is sometimes useful.

Food Preparation

Keep the reheating of food to a minimum, especially in the first stage of the Plan (while you are trying to reestablish and boost metabolic function). Enzymes are lost when food changes state, and in the case of reheating, we are going from fresh to cooked (one state), cooked to cold (a second state), and cold to reheated (a third state). By the time the food reaches the third state, there may still be some nutritional value, but there will not be any enzymes left. We really want to promote enzymes in the digestive process. You will find that freshly prepared food is best for stimu-

NOTES

lating metabolism in the initial stages of the Plan. You will be adding more raw food and less animal protein when you achieve results and you are into the second and third stages of the Plan, and gourmet reheated food will not be as much of an issue.

A Game Plan for Eating Out

Since a big part of the Plan is learning to ask for what you need and want in life—not only food but also support and acknowledgment—it is important that you learn to do this in the public domain and to be comfortable with it.

When you go out to a restaurant, check out the menu and see if there are things that will work for you. As you begin the Plan, you might even call ahead to order what you want. Most restaurants have their menus online nowadays, so you can go to the Internet and take a look beforehand if you wish. Watch for dressings, sauces, potatoes, and soups. There are so many additives and sugars in pre-prepared food, and even in regular restaurant food. Ask the wait staff questions about sauces and how the food is cooked. I have found that if you are good humored about it, most servers and kitchen staff will bend over backward to help you, after all, most of them are foodies. If you are dining at a restaurant in Europe, it is almost never an issue, as healthful, unprocessed food is almost always available at every meal. Of course, better-quality restaurants serve better-quality food. If your friends are open, let them know what you are doing and ask for support. If they are not, just make your own flow and go with it.

There are lots of options if visiting restaurants. Going to eat at someone's home is quite a different situation. During the first stages of the Plan, my clients often choose to eat beforehand and then join the others later for a cup of tea or a glass of wine. This can be an effective approach if the idea suits you. It can help you stay on course, while still allowing you to remain in good stead with your friends. When your friends see your results, they will no doubt ensure that they prepare or have food on hand that you can eat.

Salt

As previously mentioned in Chapter Six under "Refined Salt versus Unrefined Sea Salt," getting rid of all refined salt is a necessary part of the Plan. Unprocessed sea salt is the choice. Carry it with you if you often eat in restaurants or with friends. Refined table salt is one of the seven deadly sins in the case of this plan. It can cause water retention (edema), high blood pressure, and lethargy. Table salt does not enhance the taste of food; it masks it.

Making an Exception

One of the most debilitating facets of dieting is the idea of cheating. Whenever we go outside the guidelines prescribed by a particular diet, we consider this to be cheating. With this attitude, we disempower ourselves as though we were children living with a set of rules about which we have no choice. Yet the truth is, we do have choices as adults, and all we have to do is be responsible for the consequences of those choices.

I am embarrassed for people when they are eating within a system that is in support of their health and they say things like, "Oh, I just couldn't resist," "It was more than I could handle," or "I just had to have some." I am always tempted to yell in response, "Come on now, let's get real. You *could* resist. You did not *have* to do it, and it was *not* more than you could handle. You *chose* to do it!" It may be that you did it for approval, or to not stand out, or from peer pressure, but you ultimately made the choice.

We excuse ourselves by imagining we are victims of circumstance. If that is the reason that we fall off the wagon, we have disempowered ourselves totally by not taking responsibility for our choices. If we buy into our own story and just give up, where does it get us? We lose our sense of control and also some self-respect. We will continually fall prey to external excuses and make the exception into the rule. How can we shift this mental perspective and begin to empower ourselves? How can we be kind to ourselves without being too indulgent?

I have a friend in France whose father I really admire. He is such an eloquent gentleman. He is one of those true European old country gentlemen in all senses of the word, conservative but savvy. Successful in business and living by great values, Michel is truly deserving of the respect felt by his peers and family. I have met few men like him in my life. Michel, too, made a commitment to a lifestyle change involving food choices. Like everything else he does, he has had great success.

One morning when I was staying at their home in France, Michel came downstairs after we had all had a dinner with lots of wine

NOTES

and talk stretching late into the evening. Normally Michel would not have breakfast after such a night, since one of the guidelines of the Plan is that eating and partying late means no breakfast. But this day he announced, "Today, I will make an exception. I will be hunting all day and I need my breakfast." He assessed the circumstances and made a calculated decision that an exception was necessary. I respected that and I also knew that the exception would not happen often. Why? Because Michel understands how things work and how to be successful in his endeavors. He knows that if you make the exception the rule too frequently, the success you have built will fall apart, and you will not get the result you desire.

It is absolutely necessary that for the first three weeks of the Plan, you stay on it as if your life depended on it. It takes three weeks or twenty-one days to break or form a habit. After that, from time to time you may make an exception. If you make too many, though, you will not get the results you are looking for. And if this happens, no one is to blame. It is not about blame or being the victim. The results just will not occur, because your choices have not been in line with what works. If there are too many exceptions, the discipline you are building that is necessary to revitalize organ function and boost your metabolism will not occur. If you follow the Plan and do not make too many exceptions, you will be successful, and you will get results. After that, you can make an exception or two.

When your metabolism kicks in, is balanced, and becomes stable, you can add back many of the foods that were taken away at the beginning of the Plan to make it easier for your body to adjust and heal. At this point, the Plan's lifestyle falls into place and you will be in tune with your body. You will look and feel so good that anytime you go too far astray, your body will give you loud messages about what doesn't work. And you will listen! You will listen because you will know how. You will have developed the self-respect and sensitivity to want to feel as good physically, mentally, and emotionally as you have for the past six months to a year, and you will be more committed to that than to your old habits.

I think this attitude, if adopted, might change the way we view the world, *n'est-ce pas?*

Cleansing and Transition

You can refer to this summary of the important points as you progress through the first stage (Cleansing and Transition) of the Plan:

- Follow the food lists below, and use the *The Alive Recipe Collection: Sculpting Your Body with Food* cookbook.
- Have the honey-cinnamon-butter toast for breakfast every day except when on "the boil"; eat as much as you need to last until lunch. You will find that you need less as you go along.
- Eat within the designated times except for one late dinner each week:
- Breakfast: between 4 a.m. and 8 a.m.
- Lunch: between 11 a.m. and 1:30 p.m.
- Dinner: between 5 p.m. and 6:30 p.m. (stretch it to 7 if you must)
- Eat slowly and chew your food well, and eat

only one meal during each mealtime (i.e., don't have a snack at 11 a.m. and then a meal at 12:30 p.m.).

- Eat your meals until you feel comfortably full, adjusting the quantity over the first three weeks. Your stomach will tell you when you have had enough as you begin to listen to your body.
- Alternate meals daily so that starch meals and fruit meals are incorporated into your meal plans. For example, this lunch and dinner plan incorporates a starch-only meal for dinner:
  - Lunch: fish with ginger cream sauce, green beans, and salad with oil dressing.
  - Dinner: brown rice, steamed veggies with herbs and spices, and salad with oil-free dressing (Dijon mustard and cider vinegar make a nice dressing without oil).
- If you get tired or have a blood sugar drop between 3 and 4 in the afternoon, have a cup of white, green, or black tea, or a stimulating herbal tea such as ginger tea.
- Wine or beer is permitted with lunch and dinner, but only if you have substantial food in your stomach, such as meat, cheese, or olives.
- Caffeinated drinks are permitted only for those who have no problems with energy or thyroid function. These people should drink green tea, white tea, hot or cold herbal teas, hot water with lemon, or cold water with a little apple cider vinegar. The sterols in coffee inhibit the production of thyroid hormones; however, black coffee once a week is fine if you can take it.
- A drop or two of organic and/or food-grade peppermint oil can be used to assist in digestion and provide a little shot of mid-afternoon energy, as well as make your breath

NOTES

133

sweeter to both yourself and others.

- Do "the boil" as close to the third week as possible. Work it into your schedule so you have no major social engagements during this time.

- Get the food combining, chewing, and times down over the first three weeks, then start adding in the other support activities, such as breathing, loving kindness practice, dry skin brushing, The Five Tibetans, and Tibetan Acupressure.

- Gradually, over the first three weeks of the program, adopt the practice of having 4 cups (1 L) of the Cleansing and Transition Tea daily before or between meals. (Please see the Resources section.)

- At the end of the second month, add meditation or *Holosync*.

> **What's changed in the past four months? I have increased energy and haven't taken an Advil or any Maalox. Most importantly, I have regained a sense of control. I now listen to my body, and the result is a renewed sense of myself—a happier, more balanced, and healthier me.**
> — *Liz M., Advertising Executive Toronto, Canada*

ing kindness practice, the Tibetan metabolic exercises, and Tibetan Acupressure.

- After the second three-week cycle: Do "the boil" for four days.

- After two months: Have a coaching session.

- Get coaching and support throughout and/ or get a buddy to work with.

The Plan is a way of eating and living that will change the way your body processes food, metabolizes protein, and deals with sugar. It also balances hormones and provides a natural anti-inflammatory effect. As you detox and assimilate changes, you may experience physical and emotional ups and downs, as well as ups and downs in energy. Please do not rely on the scale. *Weigh yourself every two weeks— or less often or not at all if you find it depresses you.*

The Plan is not about losing weight. Weight loss will occur, just not in the way you are accustomed to losing, and it will take time. Your shape will change and you will lose cellulite, drop sizes, and gain energy. But all of your changes will not necessarily show up on the scale. Your clothes will fit differently, your body will "morph,"

Summary

- First three weeks: Practice food combining, chew properly, eat within the specified times, and drink the Alive Plan tea.

- After three weeks: Do "the boil" for four days.

- After one month: Have a coaching session.

- Second three weeks: Add breathwork, lov-

and you will like it. Dropping only fat changes your overall appearance, but on the Plan, your mental attitude will also shift and brighten. Your appetite for food and for life will be restored. Vitality will be your second name, and people will gravitate toward you.

Balance and Support

By the time you come to this stage of the program, you will have lost the weight you wanted, or you will have attained a body size and shape that you feel good about. Your metabolic rate will be humming along, your hormones will be balanced, or balancing, and your digestion will be running smoothly. In fact, you will be feeling great and ready for the next steps.

Balance and Support Steps

• Continue with the same breakfast as in the Cleansing and Transition stage.

• Continue to have your meals at the designated times, but now you can have two late evening meals a week instead of just one. You can also now have breakfast the next morning after having a late evening meal. However, if you get signals that your body does not like eating late, try to avoid it. By this point, you will be in tune with your body, and when you listen to it, you will be able to assess what works for you and what doesn't.

• Continue with your breathing and the Tibetan metabolic exercises. Raise your heart rate to a level where you break a sweat at least three times a week, and continue for at least twelve minutes to keep metabolic rate humming.

• Continue with the Cleansing and Transition Tea and the Tibetan footwork.

• Begin to change your food combining by

NOTES

adding brown rice or risotto to a fish meal once a week for three weeks. (This is sometimes better done at lunch than at dinner, as you might find it a little hard to digest protein and starches together later in the day.)

• After having rice with fish once a week for three weeks, for the next three weeks, add rice once a week to a meal that includes meat or poultry.

• You may find that you will never be able to eat bread with lunch and dinner again, and that sandwiches are off the menu. See what your body tells you, but I find most people cannot deal with bread at meals other than breakfast, unless they want to watch their weight move up and their energy falter.

• Listen to how your body responds to the changes you make. Notice how they affect your digestion. If you experience gas or bloating, or you feel sluggish or uncomfortable, go back to the way you were eating before you made the change. Remember, your body is now a lean, keen, burning machine, just like that Maserati. To keep it that way you will have to listen to the engine and manage the steering.

• After the initial six weeks of the Balance and Support stage, add back the following one by one (with a few days between each addition), but in no special order:

  • Sweet potatoes
  • Fresh fruit added to breakfast
  • Radishes and cucumber (which, according to Chinese medicine, alter hormones, so eat them infrequently)
  • Cabbage and turnip

• Beans and lentils
• Nuts

As you try these foods, you may find that some of them don't sit well with your body. You will have to make assessments about their effect by noticing the way your body responds to each food. Each body responds differently; I find that many people do not digest beans well, and very few can digest radishes. You will notice that there are foods that don't work for you and ones that do. If they don't, the discomfort may not be worth the indulgence.

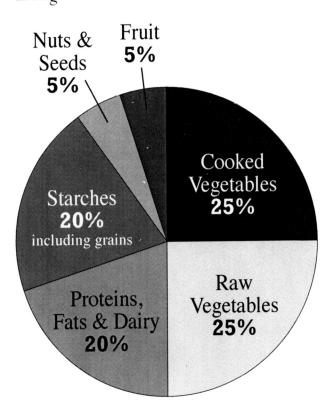

Stabilization

Congratulations! Here you are going into a totally new lifestyle with a renovated attitude, a more structured set of mind skills, a new ability for listening, and a new body to boot. I hope the Plan has given you exactly what you needed and that you are ready to continue living, loving, and eating consciously.

In order to maintain your continued success, the following are foods that you must continue to avoid as part of your new lifestyle:

- White flour, white sugar, table salt, cow's milk, soy milk, unfermented soy products, preservatives, additives, colorings, and preserved meat and fish.
- Garlic and onions. Although your taste buds will have changed, you may or may not still like them. Most people find garlic and onions too strong after having been initiated into the Plan lifestyle. Remember, too, these foods are highly stimulating, reduce concentration, and can cause hormone imbalance.
- Additionally, it is important to limit canned and packaged foods, as well as honey, sugar, molasses, maple syrup, sorghum, acacia, and stevia. Even though some of these sweeteners are natural or low on the glycemic index, they will stimulate your taste for sugar.

Here are some additional tips to help keep you on track:

- Add "the boil"! Whenever you find yourself going off track, do "the boil" for four days; it will put you back into doing things that work.
- Keep the breakfast going, it will be something that provides stability, will continue to cut your desire for sugar, and act as a daily trigger to remind you to eat well and consciously.
- Continue to follow the eating times as much as possible, and try not to eat late more than two or three times a week. Eating late every day will slow down your energy and your digestion.

NOTES

The dry skin brushing, Tibetan metabolic exercises, footwork, breathing, meditation, and loving kindness practice are practices for life. They will support the structure of your life and give you peace and satisfaction at all levels.

Happy, healthy wishes for a good life. May you have continued success, joy, and peace.

A Day in the Life of the Plan

Of course, everyone's schedule varies, but make up a plan for yourself that looks something like this. A structured life is a healthy life. You need room for flexibility, but structure and good habits always work.

A little practice that guides my days is called "The Three Noble Principles: Good in the Beginning, Good in the Middle, and Good at the End." Sound good? The first part (good in the beginning) involves being motivated and having a focus for the day. The focus could be making sure that you are kind and that your actions contribute to others in a way that reduces the suffering in their life and in yours. The good in the middle is to hold that intention or motivation during the day and be mindful and present as the day goes on. When you find yourself not being present and mindful, you forgive yourself and come back to your intentional way of being. The good at the end is to review your day before going to sleep and forgive yourself for what you did not accomplish, to acknowledge yourself for things accomplished and contributions made, and to dedicate that to the benefit of all. Sleep will be much easier when all of that is done.

Morning

The following is a suggested time for getting up. Ideally you should be able to wake up without an alarm clock. Over time, with practice, your internal clock will be set, and you will naturally awaken at whatever time you set it for.

6:30 a.m.: Wake up
- Sit up in bed and do breathing and loving kindness practice for at least two minutes
- Set your motivation for the day
- Meditate for 5 to 20 minutes

7:00 a.m.: Get out of bed
- Do the Five Tibetan Rites exercises
- Put on the kettle
- Set out your clothes for the day
- Do dry skin brushing
- Have a shower or bath and get dressed

7:30 a.m.: Breakfast
- Take supplements
- Have a cup of the Cleansing and Transition Tea
- Cook breakfast: wheat-free toast with the honey-cinnamon-butter spread, oatmeal, or wheat-free cereal with honey-cinnamon-butter spread
- Sit down and have a leisurely breakfast

8:00 a.m.: Start your busy day

10:00 a.m.: Have a mid-morning cup of Cleansing and Transition Tea or hot herbal tea

138

Midday

Between 11:00 a.m. and 1:30 p.m.
• Have a food-combined lunch
• Have the Cleansing and Transition Tea with lunch

3:00 p.m.: Have a mid-afternoon cup of the Cleansing and Transition Tea or hot herbal tea

Evening

Fit in a cardio-walk either early evening or after dinner at least three times a week.

Between 5:00 p.m. and 6:30 p.m.
• Have a food-combined dinner
• Have the Cleansing and Transition Tea with dinner

Early evening: Do the Tibetan Acupressure footwork

8:00 p.m.: Take supplements and a bedtime tea

9:30 p.m.: Get ready for bed

9:45 p.m.: Review your day, acknowledge your successes, forgive your failures, and clean the slate for the next day

10:00 p.m.: Go to bed

Do "the boil" every twenty-one days

NOTES

Waking Up to a New World View

CHAPTER TWELVE

This is the true joy of life: being used for a purpose recognized by yourself as a mighty one; being thoroughly worn out before you are thrown on a scrap heap; being a force of Nature instead of a feverish, selfish little clod of ailments and grievances, complaining that the world will not devote itself to making you happy.

— George Bernard Shaw (1856–1950)

Myths of Scarcity

Recently I was reading a book by Lynne Twist called *The Soul of Money*. It is about how our culture drives us to believe three toxic myths:

1. There's not enough.
2. More is better.

3. That is just the way it is.

These statements struck me hard, and so I share them with you now in the hope that they will crystallize some truth for you as well. In fact, I would like to conclude my book with the whole-hearted hope that in working on the Plan and living closer to your true potential you will expose and defeat these myths in your own life.

As soon as I saw these three myths listed on the page, I recognized clearly that there were many times in my life when they were running me. They are so ingrained as reality in our culture that most of us are blind to the detrimental effect they have on us. They have the power to misdirect, to dishearten, and to even defeat the spirit and rob the soul. I know for myself that there are times when I become entangled in their web of deceit.

The first myth is "there's not enough." There is not enough money, food, opportunity, time, material possessions, love, and more. I am sure you can come up with a list of things you feel are lacking in your life. This myth makes you feel powerless to do anything but suffer "the lack."

The second is "more is better." This may be especially true in the domain of assets. Striving for more is what life is about in our modern world. If you have less, it is seen as a reflection of you as a person. Our culture is driven by this principle. Lynne Twist speaks of a certain group of women, career executives in a major corporation, who work fourteen-hour days; hire people to take care of their children and homes; and are obsessed by their jobs and the race for more money, bigger houses, faster cars, trendier clothes, and better schools. All of them keep hoping that someday they will be able to take holidays and spend time with their kids. These women are driven by guilt for not doing what they know they really want to be doing. Their successes are empty.

The third myth is "that is just the way it is." This myth reflects a resignation to the idea that whatever cards you are dealt is what you have to live with. There is little hope that you could work through your condition, whether it is on the high end of the "have" circuit or the low end. As we all know, the cycle of poverty is not only in third-world countries and distant lands. It is right here in our own backyard. Welfare breeds welfare, poverty breeds poverty. And on the other end of the spectrum, wealth breeds wealth. All of it is dysfunctional, because people feel stuck and dissatisfied, whether they have or have not.

Lynne Twist was a fundraiser for the Hunger Project, a charity established in the 1970s to raise awareness of hunger and death by starvation on the planet. Its philosophy was to establish solutions that empower people to create a resolution to their own problems. The project was also created so that caring individuals could experience the sense of being able to make a difference in this worldwide condition called hunger. These people needed to know that there was a way that they could make a difference. What Lynne discovered and shared with people was that the power to make a difference globally comes from making a difference in your own life and shifting your perspective of responsibility from burden and guilt to the ability to respond.

In speaking with my friend Terry, someone who has helped me to understand the Plan in so many contexts, I realized that much of what we are dealing with in this program is eliminating that idea of scarcity. In the everyday diet paradigm, we are swamped by scarcity and limitation. In the Plan, we give ourselves permission to eat well and respond to our body's natural needs. The principles of the Plan bring us in tune with what is needed, while encouraging us to be responsible for our exceptions and to make choices wisely and with conscious awareness.

Getting back to the basics of nature and what works in eating habits is responsible action that empowers you. By empowering yourself, you become more grounded, self-sustaining, confident, and trusting. This change in perspective will transform the rest of your life into a plethora of possibilities, rather than a series of dilemmas.

When we begin to eliminate scarcity in one area of life, it starts to disappear elsewhere as well. When we relax, enjoy our food, and take care of ourselves, things slow down and we begin to let go. Time seems to expand and solutions to problems become more evident. Barriers to our well-being turn into opportunities that are actually exciting.

Are you willing to have all of your issues around scarcity clear up? Are you willing to be fully present to the joys of life and what it has to offer? And then, as part and parcel of the process, are you determined to begin to make the difference that you dream of making in your life and in the world?

If we take the energy that we tie up in our anxiety and fear over issues of scarcity and lack, and focus it instead on our vision of success, our blessings, and our love and appreciation for ourselves and others, we cannot help but succeed. We can stop listening to the myths and begin listening to our body and our own inner self. We can choose in each and every moment to let the powerful partnership we create with the Alive Plan reconnect us to a natural way of being with ourselves and with our world. We can inspire in ourselves and in others a deep commitment and a re-awakening to be the best of exactly who we are, in service to us all.

May it be of benefit.

NOTES

Food Lists

Foods You May Eat Freely

Vegetables

- Bok choy
- Avocado, celery
- Eggplant, tomatoes
- Endives, artichoke
- All green leafy vegetables, including spinach and kale
- Mushrooms of all kinds
- Zucchini, all summer squash

Note: there are many other vegetables not listed here that are complex carbohydrates, feel free to eat them as well.

Animal Protein

- Fish: grilled, poached, sautéed
- Meat (beef, lamp, pork, veal): grilled, poached, or sautéed
- Poultry: grilled, poached, or sautéed

Vegetable Protein

All seeds are permitted, including pumpkin, sunflower, sesame, and poppy; however, nuts are not permitted during the Cleansing and Transition stage, since they are difficult to digest and are often moldy. Raw almonds limited to six per day with protein meals are allowed.

Fermented and Cultured Foods

All are permitted in moderation, including fermented soy, such as tempeh, wheat-free/gluten-free tamari, and natto.

Fats and Oils

- Olive oil, flax oil, safflower oil, sesame oil, nut and seed oils (unprocessed and cold pressed)
- Butter (unsalted), preferably cultured and organic, from raw milk if possible

Vinegar

All vinegar except sweet rice vinegar and vinegars with added sugar; permitted vinegars include apple cider vinegar (preferred), balsamic, white wine vinegar, red wine vinegar, herb vinegars, and umeboshi plum vinegar.

Seasoning and Condiments

- Unprocessed sea salt
- Umeboshi plum, Dijon mustard, capers, olives
- Fresh or dried herbs
- Hot spices are permitted, *but not in excess*

Cultured Vegetables and Sprouted Grains and Seeds

Cultured vegetables, such as sauerkraut, and sprouted grains and seeds of all kinds are permitted for those who can tolerate traces of gluten. For those who have celiac disease or are gluten-intolerant, only sprouted gluten-free grains and sprouted seeds and beans are permitted.

Dairy

Cultured milk products such as yogurt, *fromage blanc*, and plain kefir, with no added sugar; cow's milk cheese for those who tolerate it; goat's and sheep's milk cheeses are preferred.

Fruit (three times a week only)

- Ripe bananas as a meal (as many as you want), whole, mashed, or as part of a smoothie using ice and spice only (add berries if desired)
- Berries: all kinds sliced or made into a smoothie with ice and spice
- Grapefruit: used to flavor meat, fish, or in hot water to drink between meals; may also be eaten as a meal or as an appetizer
- Lemon or lime: used to flavor meat, fish, or in hot water to drink

Fruit Compote

Use fruit such as apples, plums, cherries, apricots, and pears, but no tropical fruits such as pineapple, mango, or papaya until you get to the Balancing and Stabilization sections of the Plan.

Sample Fruit Compote

Fruit compote is used during "the boil" part of the Plan. For a smoother texture, you can blend the compote in a food processor before serving.

Yield: 2 to 4 servings

6 apples, cored and peeled
6 pears, cored and peeled
6 apricots, pitted
1 handful of blueberries
1 handful of raspberries
1 cup (250 mL) water
1 fruit tea bag
¼–½ teaspoon (1–2.5 mL) ground cinnamon or cardamom (optional)

Place the apples, pears, apricots, and berries in a medium heavy-bottomed saucepan and bring slowly to a boil over medium-high heat. Reduce the heat to low and simmer for 20 minutes, or until the fruit is tender.

Meanwhile, bring the water to a boil in a small saucepan, add the tea bag, and let steep for a few minutes. Remove the tea bag and add the flavored water to the fruit. Stir in the cinnamon or cardamom if desired, and serve.

NOTES

Foods You May Eat Three Times a Week

- Boiled potatoes (no oil or butter) with vegetables is allowed as a meal
- Broccoli, cauliflower
- Carrots, beets
- Cheese
- Corn on the cob (as much as you like) with salt only, no butter, may be eaten with vegetables; you may have corn and potatoes together
- Cream (heavy), crème fraîche

- Eggs
- Pâté
- Fresh sweet green peas
- Yellow beans

Foods You Are *Required* to Eat Three Times a Week

- Brown rice pasta, quinoa pasta, or soba (buckwheat) pasta with fresh vegetables (no butter or oil) *or* boiled brown rice with vegetables (no butter or oil)
- Separation of heavy protein and light starches is important to aid the process; starch meals must be on alternating days

Foods You May *Not* Eat at Any Time during the Cleansing and Transition Part of the Plan

- Asparagus
- Beans and lentils
- Black and white pepper
- Bread (except wheat-free bread at breakfast)
- Cabbage (except sauerkraut)
- Canned or prepared food (except tomatoes, artichokes, capers, and olives)
- Cucumbers (pickled are permitted)
- Deep-fried foods
- Distilled alcohol and liquor (wine and beer with food are fine)
- Fresh fruit (except lemon, grapefruit, bananas, and berries)
- Garlic and onions
- Juice (may have fresh vegetable juice)
- Malt sugar (or any kind of processed sugar products, or any food containing any of

these)
- Milk (animal, soy, or other)
- Nuts (permitted for vegetarians)
- Pickles (unless with vinegar and spice only)
- Pop, soda (mineral water is fine)
- Processed or deli-style meat or fish
- Processed or hydrogenated oils, fats, or margarine
- Radishes (unless pickled or cultured)
- Smoked fish or meat
- Soy (fermented products are okay; e.g., tempeh, wheat-free/gluten-free tamari)
- Wheat and wheat gluten products
- Sugar and sugar substitutes of all kinds (honey at breakfast is fine)
- Sweet potatoes, melons (for the Cleansing and Transition part of the Plan)
- Turnip (for the Cleansing and Transition part of the Plan)
- White flour, table salt

Permitted Beverages

- Beer (lager and ale) and red or white wine and champagne are permitted (make sure you have a reasonable amount of food in your stomach before imbibing)
- Unflavored coffee (you may add a piece of lemon zest to reduce the acidity of coffee or black tea) **Caution**: if you have a thyroid dysfunction, limit your coffee intake
- Tea: black, green, and herbal teas and water can be enjoyed freely
- It is advisable to drink fluids between meals only; wine, beer, or sips of water, tea, or coffee may be drunk during meals

NOTES

Food Combining Chart

LIST A
Proteins
All Meat
All Poultry
Fish
Eggs
Seeds
(Nuts in later phases
of food plan)

LIST B
Neutral Foods
Most Vegetables
(except high starch)
Most Salads & Herbs

LIST C
Fats & Dairy
Heavy Cream
Cultured Butter (no salt)
Cheeses
Olive Oil, Flax Oil,
Seed Oils
(cold-pressed,
unprocessed)

LIST D
Starches
No Wheat
Only Fermented
Soy Products
Wheat-free or Rye Bread
Wheat-free Pasta
Potatoes and Corn
Brown Rice

LIST E
Fruit - Seasonal
Citrus permitted,
except Oranges

Mix anything from List A with Lists B and C.
Never mix Lists A and C with List D.
List E: Fruit is always by itself, as a meal.

Bibliography

Ackerman, Jennifer. *Sex Sleep Eat Drink Dream: A Day in the Life of Your Body*. New York: Houghton Mifflin, 2007.

Batmanghelidj, F. *Your Body's Many Cries for Water*, 2nd ed. Vienna, VA: Global Health Solutions, 2003.

Brownstein, David. *Overcoming Thyroid Disorders*, 2nd ed. West Bloomfield, MI: Medical Alternative Press, 2002.

———. *Salt: Your Way to Health*, 2nd ed. West Bloomfield, MI: Medical Alternative Press, 2006.

Cameron, Julia. *The Artist's Way: A Spiritual Path to Higher Creativity*. New York: Tarcher/ Putnam, 1992.

Childre, Doc, and Howard Martin, with Donna Beech. *The HeartMath Solution: The Institute of HeartMath's Revolutionary Program for Engaging the Power of the Heart's Intelligence*. San Francisco: HarperCollins, 1999.

D'Adamo, Peter J., with Catherine Whitney. *Eat Right 4 Your Type: The Individualized Diet Solution to Staying Healthy, Living Longer & Achieving Your Ideal Weight*. New York: G. P. Putnam's Sons, 1996.

Daniel, Kaayla T. *The Whole Soy Story: The Dark Side of America's Favorite Health Food*. Washington, DC: New Trends Publishing, 2005.

Diamond, Harvey and Marilyn. *Fit for Life*. New York: Warner Books, 1985.

Dooley, Mike. *Notes from the Universe: New Perspectives from an Old Friend*. New York: Simon & Schuster, 2007.

Fallon, Sally. *Nourishing Traditions: The Cookbook that Challenges Politically Correct Nutrition and the Diet Dictocrats*, 2nd edition. Washington, DC: New Trends Publishing, 1999.

Fuhrman, Joel. *Eat to Live: The Revolutionary Formula for Fast and Sustained Weight Loss*. New York: Little, Brown and Company, 2003.

Gerber, Richard. *Vibrational Medicine: The #1 Handbook of Subtle-Energy Therapies*, 3rd ed. Rochester, VT: Inner Traditions, Bear & Company, 2001.

Gunaratana, Bhante Henepola. *Mindfulness in Plain English*, 2nd ed. Somerville, MA: Wisdom Publications, 2002.

Habgood, Jackie. *The Hay Diet Made Easy: A Practical Guide to Food Combining*. London, UK: Souvenir Press, 1997.

Harris, Bill. *Thresholds of the Mind: Your Personal Roadmap to Success, Happiness, and Contentment*. Beaverton, OR: Centerpointe Research Institute, 2002.

Kelder, Peter, and J. W. Watt, ed. *The Eye of Revelation: The Ancient Tibetan Rites of Rejuvenation*. Online: Booklocker.com, 2008.

Kilham, Christopher S. *The Five Tibetans: Five Dynamic Exercises for Health, Energy, and Personal Power*. Rochester, VT: Healing Arts Press, 1994.

Lama, Dalai. *Ethics for a New Millennium*. New York: Riverhead Books, 1999.

Lama, Dalai, and Howard C. Cutler. *The Art of Happiness: A Handbook for Living*. London, UK: Riverhead Books, 1998.

Linn, Denise. *Soul Coaching: 28 Days to Discover Your Authentic Self*. Carlsbad, CA: Hay House, 2003.

Maté, Gabor. *When the Body Says No: Exploring the Stress-Disease Connection*. Hoboken, NJ: John Wiley & Sons, 2011.

Mann, John, and Lar Short. *The Body of Light: History and Practical Techniques for Awakening Your Subtle Body*. Boston: Charles E. Tuttle Co., 1990.

Merton, Thomas. *The Seven Storey Mountain: An Autobiography of Faith*. Orlando, FL: Harcourt Brace & Company, 1948.

———. *Contemplative Prayer*. New York: Doubleday, 1996.

Bibliography

Meyerowitz, Steve. *Food Combining and Digestion: 101 Ways to Improve Digestion*. Great Barrington, MA: Sproutman Publications, 2002.

Nelson, Portia. *There's a Hole in My Sidewalk: The Romance of Self-Discovery*. Hillsboro, OR: Beyond Words Publishing, 1993.

Northrup, Christiane. *Women's Bodies, Women's Wisdom: Creating Physical and Emotional Health and Healing*. New York: Bantam Books, 2010.

Pollan, Michael. *In Defense of Food: An Eater's Manifesto*. New York: Penguin, 2008.

———. *The Ominivore's Dilemma: A Natural History of Four Meals*. New York: Penguin, 2006.

Price, Weston A. *Nutrition and Physical Degeneration*, 6th edition. La Mesa, CA: Price-Pottenger Nutrition Foundation, 2000.

Rinpoche, Sogyal. *The Tibetan Book of Living and Dying*. Edited by Patrick Gaffney and Andrew Harvey. San Francisco: HarperCollins, 2002.

Rinpoche, Tsoknyi. *Carefree Dignity: Discourses on Training in the Nature of Mind*. Translated by Erik Pema Kunsang and Marcia Binder Schmidt. Hong Kong: Rangjung Yeshi Publications, 1998.

Rinpoche, Yongey Mingyur. *Joyful Wisdom: Embracing Change and Finding Freedom*. Translated by Eric Swanson. New York: Three Rivers Press, 2010.

Robbins, John. *Diet for a New America: How Your Food Choices Affect Your Health, Happiness, and the Future of Life on Earth*. Tiburon, CA: H J Kramer, 1987.

———. *The Food Revolution: How Your Diet Can Help Save Your Life and Our World*. San Francisco: Conari Press, 2001.

Twist, Lynne, with Teresa Barker. *The Soul of Money: Transforming Your Relationship with Money and Life*. New York: W. W. Norton, 2003.

Weil, Andrew. *8 Weeks to Optimum Health: A Proven Program for Taking Full Advantage of Your Body's Natural Healing Power*. New York: Random House, 1997.

Witt, Carolinda. *The 10-Minute Rejuvenation Plan: T5T: The Revolutionary Exercise Program That Restores Your Body and Mind*. Mill Valley, CA: Random House, 2007.

Resources

The Alive Plan Resources:
• Coaching, support, supplements, books, tea, newsletter, video: www.aliveanenergyplanforlife.com

Alkaline Water:
• Ion Ways: www.jupiterathena.com

Biodynamic Farming:
• Products: Foxhollow Farm, Kentucky: www.foxhollow.com
• About biodynamic farming: Demeter-International: www.demeter.net

Body Care Products:
• Peppermint and other soaps, dry skin brushes: Rainbow Blossom Natural Food Market: www.rainbowblossom.com
• Makeup and skin care from Switzerland: Arbonne, Eunice Ray, National Director: www.arbonne.com

Breathing and Meditation:
• Nooma #14, Breathe, DVD, by Rob Bell: www.christianbook.com
• Tsoknyi Rinpoche, Pundarika Foundation, meditation and retreats: www.pundarika.org
• Sogyal Rinpoche, Rigpa, meditation practice retreats: www.rigpa.org

Celtic Sea Salt:
• Selina Naturally: www.selinanaturally.com
• Rainbow Blossom Natural Food Markets: www.rainbowblossom.com

Cleansing and Transition Tea and Infusion:
www.aliveanenergyplanforlife.com

Coaching for the Plan:
www.aliveanenergyplanforlife.com

Food:
• Rainbow Blossom Natural Food Markets: www.rainbowblossom.com
• Other natural food stores, farmer's markets, and local co-ops

Five Tibetan Rites:
Carolinda Witt:
• DVDs for easy learning: www.t5t.com/DVDs
• Training Courses: www.t5t.com/courses.php
Ellen Wood:
• "The RIGHT Way" on YouTube www.youtube.com/watch?v=HjtslbrFbLY

HeartMath:
- For international licensed HeartMath providers: www.heartmath.com
- Licensed HeartMath provider and Wellness Coach in Louisville, Kentucky: Kimberly May: 502-593-9017; inspirewell@gmail.com

High-Vitamin Butter Oil:
- Green Pasture Products: www.greenpasture.org/public/Home/index.cfm

Holistic Practitioner:
- Dr. David Brownstein (see his books on thyroid dysfunction, salt, and other alternative approaches to healing): www.drbrownstein.com

Holosync:
- Centerpointe Research Institute: www.centerpointe.com

Natural Hormone Therapy:
- American Holistic Medical Association for medical doctors, naturopathic doctors, or alternative practitioners who can prescribe natural hormone therapy: www.holisticmedicine.org

Organize Your Space:
- Arin Stodin, StodinStyle, www.stowedinstyle.com, arinstodin@yahoo.com, 502-377-7299

Sprouting:
www.rainbowblossom.com

Soul Coaching:
www.soul-coaching.com
- Jenn de Valk, Salt Spring Island, BC, Canada
- Patti Allen, Toronto, ON, Canada
- Michelle Chant, Canberra, ACT, Australia

Soul of Money Institute:
www.soulofmoney.org

Sullivan University College of Pharmacy:
www.sullivan.edu/pharmacy

Tibetan Acupressure System:
- Rae's foot self-care video demo: www.youtube.com/selfcareforthefeet
- Acupressure video demo: www.tibetan-acupressure.com

Yoga:
- Moksha yoga:
  Canada: www.mokshayoga.ca
  US: www.mokshayogauptown.com
- Betsy's Hot Yoga, Louisville, Kentucky: www.hotyogalouisville.com
- New Zealand: www.hotyogaasylimb.co.nz

NOTES

Index

CPSIA information can be obtained at www.ICGtesting.com
Printed in the USA
LVOW021251081211

258342LV00003B/2/P